The Infertility
Companion *for*
Catholics

"For a couple desiring children, discovering their infertility can be devastating. This personal witness of two couples' faith journey struggling with infertility is uplifting and refreshing. This labor of love is also extremely well researched and solidly within the teaching of the Catholic Church. Highly recommended!"

Rev. Alfred Cioffi
Senior Fellow
National Catholic Bioethics Center

"The suffering of infertility is an especially painful participation in the cross of Jesus Christ. In this thoughtful guide, the authors provide a spiritual roadmap for walking through this suffering in obedience to the call of our Lord. This book provides both hope and solace to Catholic spouses who seek to follow Jesus and to be faithful to his teachings as expressed by the Church."

Angela Franks
Director of Theology Programs
Theological Institute for the New Evangelization
Saint John's Seminary

"*The Infertility Companion* is a sensitive, thought-provoking reflection on the effect of infertility in the lives of couples who experience it. It is a beautiful blend of Church teaching, spirituality, and personal testimony. A must-read for couples having difficulty conceiving and for those who love them!"

Steven Bozza
Director
Respect Life Office
Archdiocese of Philadelphia

"In a genre where both Christian and secular books abound, we are so blessed to finally have a resource that is authentically Catholic! *The Infertility Companion for Catholics* provides a well-thought-out, comprehensive, and sensitive manual for Catholic couples struggling with the difficult cross of infertility."

Laura Flaherty
Founder
Hannah's Heart Catholic Infertility Support Group

"This book provides excellent insights on physical realities, moral implications, psychological ramifications, and Church teachings related to infertility. It is a much-needed resource, and I will recommend it to the many couples who turn to Elizabeth Ministry for guidance."

Jeannie Hannemann
International Founder
Elizabeth Ministry

"Sharing the latest in advanced diagnostic treatment options that fall within the teachings of the Magisterium and providing faith-filled tools for both partners, the authors have created the perfect primer for married couples facing the stress, heartbreak, and uncertainty of infertility. Also a fantastic resource for family members, friends, and pastoral staff who share this difficult path with infertile couples. Let this book help strengthen your marriage and your spiritual life."

Lisa M. Hendey
Author of *A Book of Saints for Catholic Moms*

"A guiding light to infertile couples wishing to learn more about treatment options in light of the Church's teaching, and how to address this suffering emotionally and spiritually. Offers great inner consolation, as it addresses the difficult topics of infertility, discernment, miscarriage, and adoption. A must-read for infertile couples!"

Marie Meaney
Author of *Embracing the Cross of Infertility*

The Infertility Companion *for* Catholics

Spiritual
and
Practical
Support
for Couples

Angelique Ruhi-López and
Carmen Santamaría

Foreword by John and Claire Grabowski

Members of the Pontifical Council for the Family

ave maria press AMP notre dame, indiana

Imprimatur: Most Reverend Thomas G. Wenski
Archbishop of Miami
Given at Miami, Florida, on November 4, 2011

Founded in 1865, Ave Maria Press is a ministry of the United States Province of Holy Cross.

www.avemariapress.com

Paperback: ISBN-10 1-59471-289-1   ISBN-13 978-1-59471-289-0

E-book: ISBN-10 1-59471-344-8   ISBN-13 978-1-59471-344-6

Cover image © Istock Images.

Cover and text design by Katherine Robinson Coleman.

Printed and bound in the United States of America.

Library of Congress Cataloging-in-Publication Data

Ruhi-López, Angelique.

The infertility companion for Catholics: spiritual and practical support for couples / Angelique Ruhi- López and Carmen Santamaría.

p. cm.

ISBN 978-1-59471-289-0 (pbk.) -- ISBN 1-59471-289-1 (pbk.)

1. Infertility--Religious aspects--Catholic Church. 2. Human reproductive technology--Religious aspects--Catholic Church. I. Santamaría, Carmen. II. Title.

RC889.R897 2012

616.6'92--dc23

2011044924

Contents

Foreword

"Behold, children are a gift from the Lord" declared the Psalmist (Ps 127:3), and undoubtedly, most couples would agree. In our twenty-six years of marriage many of our greatest blessings—and, at times, greatest challenges—have come from the five children with whom we have been blessed by the Author of Life. Couples who face the challenge of infertility are profoundly aware of this gift of children through its absence from their lives.

While we have not had to contend with infertility in our own marriage, years of working in various marriage-related ministries (preparation, support, teaching, and writing) have brought us into contact with many couples whose lives and marriages have been touched by this cross. Working with and listening to such couples through the years has led us to remark many times that the Church community can and should do more to offer its support to those whose longing for children remains unfulfilled.

It is precisely for this need that *The Infertility Companion for Catholics: Spiritual and Practical Support for Couples* by Angelique Ruhi-López and Carmen Santamaría offers a unique and valuable contribution. The authors describe the book as a companion for those contending with the challenges of infertility as faithful Catholics. While aimed in a particular way at infertile couples, the book offers a helpful perspective to anyone seeking to understand this challenge more deeply and support those living with it.

The book is also written in an engaging and accessible style. The authors share not only their research on the subject, but their own experiences as women who have faced the challenge of infertility for significant periods of their married lives. As a result, some chapters are coauthored and some are written by Angelique, others by Carmen. One chapter was written by Carmen's husband to provide a male perspective on infertility. Testimony from the experiences of other infertile couples is woven through the work. The result is a book that is at once bracingly candid and profoundly hopeful.

But it would be a mistake to view *The Infertility Companion for Catholics* as some kind of self-help or group therapy text for the infertile. The book contains a wealth of information on infertility, current medical treatments, the fertility industry, the impact of infertility on women and men, its impact on marriage, miscarriage, and the many facets of the decision to adopt. Many chapters conclude with lists of additional resources for topics treated—helpful glossaries, discussion points, print resources, websites, blogs, and educational and support groups. Yet the information is always presented in an accessible and user-friendly fashion so that the reader is never overloaded.

The authors do more than provide information about the phenomenon of infertility. One of the great strengths of the book is that it seeks to faithfully present the teaching of the Church on the subject. Angelique Ruhi-López and Carmen Santamaría provide clear overviews of procedures which the Church opposes, procedures which the Church supports, and cases where there is still theological debate. But more than this, they highlight the great service the Church provides in defending the dignity of the human person, the gift of children, and the inseparable connection between the unitive and procreative meanings of sex. The teaching of the Church can enable couples to work their way through the bewildering array of complex medical treatments and competing voices offering advice to discern those practices that enable infertile persons to care for both their bodies and their souls. As Pope Benedict XVI has reminded us: "To defend the truth, to articulate it with humility and conviction, and to bear witness to it in life are therefore exacting and indispensable forms of charity" (*Caritas in veritate*, no. 1). This book offers precisely that profound kind of charity.

This observation points to a final strength of the book—it not only seeks to direct its reader to faithfully understand and apply the Church's teachings—it seeks to build up and support the faith of those who read it. Each chapter ends with a prayer specific to the subject treated, lending a meditative quality to the work. The authors also cite biblical examples, the saints, and great writers from the Church's spiritual tradition, particularly the Spiritual Exercises of Saint Ignatius of Loyola. This is an especially valuable resource for couples striving to maintain their prayer lives in the midst of the pain and desolation of infertility and attempting to discern options for how to move forward together. This pragmatic spirituality bears fruit in a particularly helpful discussion which treats the decision to adopt as a call separate from the recognition of infertility.

Suffering is a part of every life and every marriage. In equipping couples to face the very intense and personal cross of suffering in the form of infertility, *The Infertility Companion for Catholics* is a genuinely unique work. It is not just another book—but is, as the title suggests, a companion. Like the angel Raphael who accompanies Tobias in the book of Tobit, the work instructs, supports, guides, and encourages on a difficult journey. It is our hope that its readers will profit from its hopeful presence and wise counsel.

John and Claire Grabowski
Member Couple
The Pontifical Council for the Family

Preface

Trust in the Lord with all your heart,
on your own intelligence rely not;
In all your ways be mindful of him,
and he will make straight your paths.

Proverbs 3:5–6

Fifteen years ago, we sat on a bus and chatted nonstop during a four-hour ride home in the middle of the night after our high school's senior-class trip. Little did we know that this conversation—in which with youthful idealism we talked about our families, our plans for the future, and our common Catholic faith—would change us from acquaintances to lifelong friends.

Though we were companions on a different kind of journey at the time, God providentially cemented our friendship as he knew we would share in many other journeys together: graduations and celebrations, first jobs and first dates, breakups and breakdowns, weddings and funerals, and vacations and vocations.

Of all of our shared life experiences, it is perhaps infertility that has been the most complex and formative for us, not only as friends, but also as Catholics. We are eternally grateful to God for giving us the gift of each other as spiritual companions on this life-altering journey of infertility.

We invite you to consider this book just such a companion, as a friend that you can consult and rely on when you need to be challenged, encouraged, and understood. This companion is intended to provide moral and spiritual support as well as clear guidance on the many options that infertile couples face and how to make necessary choices while remaining faithful to the teachings of the magisterium. Its purpose is to give voice to the reality of infertility among those who seek to live as faithful Catholics.

We are proud that the Catholic Church has stood firm in defending our human dignity with respect to infertility treatments. Even people from other faith traditions who are not comfortable with potentially immoral treatment options are looking to the Catholic Church because it is one of the few religious voices to speak out and provide clear guidance in defense of human dignity and the dual unitive and procreative purposes of sex.

We have attempted to discuss the issues most relevant to Catholic couples bearing this cross. These include but are not limited to an introduction to infertility and Assisted Reproductive Technology (ART), what the Church teaches on these technologies and the hopeful medical alternatives it offers, and how to make wise decisions when pursuing treatment. The aforementioned subjects comprise the first four chapters of the book and are co-written by both of us to lay the groundwork for the emotional and spiritual sides of infertility described in chapters 5 through 12. The latter chapters include, among other things, reflections on how the infertility journey can bear spiritual fruit, tools to strengthen marriages, discerning the call to adoption, and tips for family and friends who seek to support couples experiencing infertility. Because these chapters include details unique to each of our experiences, Angelique wrote chapters 5, 7, 11, and 12; Carmen wrote chapters 4, 6, 8, and 10; and Alex, Carmen's husband, wrote chapter 9 to offer the male perspective on infertility. Each chapter also concludes with a prayer asking the Lord to walk with us as we traverse this unknown territory.

The experiences, feelings, and reflections in this book come from our individual experiences with infertility. Angelique will share how she and her husband, Richard, experienced infertility when they tried to conceive their first child. Infertility came as a surprise for them since they never had any reason to believe they would not conceive quickly. God gently reminded them that it was all in his timing. They researched what the Church teaches about Assisted Reproductive Technology (ART) and were humbled to see how deeply the Church cares for the dignity of each human person. Despite the beauty of Church teaching, the pain of infertility persisted, and Angelique longed for a resource that not only provided answers on the Church's view on acceptable treatments but also offered encouragement and hope. Thus, the idea for this book was born before her children were. Prayer and discernment led them to adopt their first son internationally after experiencing over one year of infertility. They later had three biological children as well.

Carmen and her husband, Alex, continue to struggle with the cross of infertility today. Their journey through a multitude of tests and diagnoses for the past three years has challenged and strengthened their marriage. The desire to follow God's will has given purpose to their difficulties and has helped them take comfort in their faith. They are currently finalizing the adoption of twins and hope that, by inviting readers to share in their journey, others will find companionship and peace.

In addition to sharing our own experiences, we interviewed other Catholic couples who have experienced infertility or miscarriage, and we recount some of their reflections in this book as well.

Some couples reading this companion will already have some sort of infertility diagnosis. Others may be beginning to question why it is taking so long to conceive and are curious as to how the Church can help. Please know that this book is not intended to provide diagnostic help and should not replace medical advice. Diagnoses and treatments are discussed only briefly. We encourage you to seek medical help if you suspect infertility.

Maybe you are not on the journey personally, but you wish to support a family member or friend by learning a little bit about what infertility is like. On behalf of those suffering silently, thank you for taking the time to learn about this journey and help us bear this cross.

Though we often express our raw emotions and painful experiences with infertility, our intent is never to criticize or judge others who have made or will make different choices. The feelings we express are our own and are shared so that others who are facing infertility and seeking to follow Church teaching may know they are not alone and that there are constructive ways of approaching these decisions and dealing with the powerful feelings surrounding them.

However, we do hope to challenge those who are discerning which path to take by explaining why the Catholic Church teaches as it does. We understand that what we say in this book is not necessarily popular, but we encourage you to have an open heart and mind. There have certainly been times when we both questioned the Church's teaching on these issues, but through prayer, humility, and understanding, we have come to recognize God's love and wisdom in his Church's guidance. Our prayer is that this book will do the same for you. Allow the Lord to surprise you and change your heart. "I will give you a new heart and place a new spirit within you, taking from your bodies your stone hearts and giving you natural hearts. I will put my spirit within you and make you live by my statutes, careful to observe my decrees" (Ez 36:26–27).

We invite you to join our online community at www.catholicinfertilityjourney.com, where we share experiences, resources, and prayer requests with one another. We would love to hear from you.

Acknowledgments

We are blessed to have had companions not only on our infertility journeys but also as we wrote this book.

To our loving heavenly Father, his beloved Son, and the Spirit that unites them, we are indebted for the inspiration and the perseverance to write what we hope are your words. Thank you for the vocabulary and the courage to share our difficult journey with the humble hope that it may serve others. We pray that it is pleasing to you, Lord, and to your Blessed Mother, who is our model and protectress.

We would also like to thank the staff at Ave Maria Press, especially our editor Kristi McDonald, who championed this manuscript and believed in the importance of its subject. Robert Hamma also encouraged these first-time authors and trusted us to transmit this message for faithful Catholics. Amanda Williams and all the marketing staff, as well as Jared Dees in web development, were always helpful and willing to answer our questions. Many thanks to all of you—you are consummate professionals and a joy to work with!

Nora Gonzalez and Claudia Rodriguez, our sisters in the Lord, thank you for your support, encouragement, and friendship.

We are also grateful for the prayers and support of our friends and communities, including Alas de Cristo Christian Life Community, Marriages in Victory at St. Timothy Parish, and Camino del Matrimonio. Thanks for your enthusiasm along the way. While striving to live counter-culturally, we are grateful to have been affirmed and understood by you.

We interviewed several women and couples to gain their perspectives on infertility. Aileen and Raul Escarpio, Anais and Ivan Ospina, Zilkia and Andres Jimenez, Karla and Mike Hernandez, Jessica Martinez, and Eva Gonzalez: we are blessed by your friendship, moved by your stories, and grateful for your willingness to relive tough experiences so that others may be enriched.

We also wish to thank Lourdes Santamaría-Wheeler and Martha Rodriguez for the great promotional pictures.

Angelique would like to thank:

Richard, thank you for your quiet strength and steadfast support. How humbled I am that God chose you for me and our family. There is no one else with whom I could have weathered the storm of infertility. I love you more than I can express and am grateful for you every day.

Emmanuel, Sebastian, Madeleine, and Anabella: thank you for your patience while I spent many hours writing. Thank you for always asking how the book was going and for praying for me and your Tia Carmen so earnestly. You inspire me to be a better person and to model your child-like faith. Los quiero mucho.

Many thanks to all of my amazing family for your support, prayers, and encouragement. I would especially like to thank Dad, Mom, Joaquin, Julia, Hilda, Pepe, Adrian, Naty, Isabel, Liz, Anay, Enrique, Cristy, Henry, and Bianca for taking care of the kids while I wrote—¡Gracias! Que Dios se los repague.

Carmen, you were the engine behind this book. I know that writing this while experiencing the raw emotions of infertility was not easy. Thank you for sacrificing your own comfort so that others may be comforted. I am always inspired by you and in awe of your tremendous faith. I thank God for giving us the opportunity to journey in faith through the rain and the rainbows with Him as our big yellow umbrella.

Carmen would like to thank:

Alex, thank you for believing in me and supporting me unceasingly. Not only did you encourage me, but you did what

I know was so hard for you to do. Words fail in my efforts to thank you, so I ask God to let you know how incredible you are.

Monica, thank you for your prayers that our words would be God's. May you always value your feminine genius.

Antonio Javier, thank you for letting Mami be on the computer so much without complaining. For knowing the libro was important. May you continue growing in God's grace.

Victoria and Daniel—the double blessing along this journey. I thank God for the gift of your lives and cherish the privilege of raising you.

Antonio and Marcia Iglesias, my parents, thank you for teaching me to love the Church. You have always been models of disciples living out your baptismal call. Mami, thank you for being prophetic and inspiring me to do the same.

Miriam and Inocente Santamaría gracias por el apoyo.

Angelique, your vision for this book started this work; thank you for including me in this effort. Thank you for lending me your umbrella and walking with me in the rain. Your unconditional love for my family and me is a gift for which I constantly thank God. May you continue to let God use you for his greater glory.

Ad majorem Dei gloriam
Miami, Florida
November 25, 2011

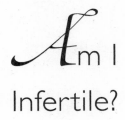m I
Infertile?

We are not human beings that have a spiritual experience.
We are spiritual beings having a human experience.

Pierre Teilhard de Chardin

One of the most difficult challenges of our journeys with infertility was coming to terms with the fact that we were possibly infertile. A few months of unsuccessful attempts to conceive left us confused: was our failure to conceive due to underlying medical issues or simply God's timing? Angelique shares how she and her husband first realized that God's plan for their family was not necessarily the same as their own:

> Paris is my absolute favorite city, and thanks to our knowl-edge of Natural Family Planning (NFP),[1] we figured out that I would be ovulating while we were there on a Euro-pean tour in 2005. We had already been trying to conceive for a few months with no success and had not been as stringent about postponing pregnancy even prior to that,

so I thought maybe we were meant to bring home a little souvenir from Paris.

Getting my period about two weeks after returning from Europe was the first really painful moment in what would become more than one year of struggling with infertility. The sadness I felt that month was not because we had not conceived in Paris (in hindsight, that doesn't seem so important anymore). It was because that was the point at which we started to realize that having children was not going to be as easy as we had anticipated and that, ultimately, we were not in control. Within a couple of months we found ourselves beginning the process of learning about infertility.

What Is Infertility?

The Centers for Disease Control and Prevention (CDC) reports that about 7.1 million women between ages 15 and 44 in the United States are considered to have "impaired fecundity," which is characterized by the CDC as the inability to conceive after one year of unprotected intercourse. According to this definition, about one in six couples is considered infertile. This includes both married and unmarried women as well as those having problems carrying a baby to term.[3] About 7.4 percent of married women ages 15 to 44 are infertile (ie, who are not surgically sterile, have not used contraception in the past twelve months, and have not become pregnant). Of that same age group, about 7.3 million have sought fertility services at some point, including medical advice, medical help to prevent miscarriage, diagnostic tests on the woman and/or man, and ovulation drugs and Assisted Reproductive Technology (ART).[4]

On one hand, these statistics tell us that we are not alone in our struggle with infertility, and that is comforting. On the other hand, it's sad to see that so many others are suffering from this too. Carmen shares how she and her husband felt when they realized they were infertile:

I don't remember an exact moment when we realized we were infertile. Having secondary infertility made it harder to come to this realization because we kept thinking we would get pregnant since we had done so successfully before.[5] Then again, maybe a part of me always foresaw or anticipated some difficulty because I remember talking to my mother before even trying to conceive about what I would do if we couldn't get pregnant. As the months went by, I started to get anxious, so I grabbed a book on infertility and started reading. This was my first concrete step on what would become a long and challenging journey.

What Causes Infertility?

About a third of the time, infertility can be traced to a cause within the woman. In another third of cases, it is the man who faces infertility. The rest of the time, it is because both partners have infertility issues or because no cause is found.[6] However, there is no single cause of infertility because a successful pregnancy is a multistep chain of events. To put it simply, achieving pregnancy includes the following steps: A woman's ovaries must be able to release a viable egg, which then must be capable of traveling down the fallopian tube. The man must be able to ejaculate, and his sperm must be able to travel to the fallopian tube. The sperm and egg must unite to fertilize the egg. And the fertilized egg must implant inside the uterus and be nurtured by the body to allow the fetus to develop and grow until it is ready for birth. Problems with any of these steps can mean infertility.[7] Given all the above factors that must work properly in order for conception to occur, combined with the need for adequate hormone levels and proper physiology, it is a miracle women ever get pregnant at all.

The modern increase in the incidence of infertility may be due to any number of reasons or perhaps a combination of reasons: Couples are having children at a later age than previous generations (the proportion of first births to women aged

30 and older has increased more than fourfold since 1975, from 5 to 24 percent in 2006).[8] Prolonged use of hormonal contraception, various environmental influences, genetic disorders, increased levels of stress, and additional sexually transmitted diseases could all be contributing factors. In short, there are many theories surrounding the cause of higher infertility rates today, but there are no definitive answers.

Female Infertility

Carmen shares her experience of finding a medical diagnosis for her infertility:

> After one year of trying to conceive, I finally had some blood work done and discovered I was hypothyroid. My doctor was convinced that this was the cause of my infertility. I began taking a pill to regulate my thyroid levels, but we still did not conceive. We went to another doctor at this point, and by now my husband was more involved because the time lapse since our first pregnancy indicated that things were certainly different this time around. This doctor looked at my NFP charts and said I had a luteal phase deficiency (meaning that the period of time in a woman's menstrual cycle between ovulation and the possible implantation of an embryo was too short and could potentially impede an embryo from properly implanting) and thus prescribed progesterone suppositories. He was very positive, and I remember feeling like we had found the solution; I was so sure we were going to get pregnant right after I started the medication. The answers seemed to fit and were relatively easy to fix so we thought everything would be fine. However, this was not the answer either, and I think the fact that my husband and I had so much hope was one of the hardest parts of the journey.

Although this is by no means an exhaustive list, below are the leading causes of infertility in women[9]:

- **Endometriosis**—occurs when the uterine tissue implants and grows outside of the uterus, often affecting the function of the ovaries, uterus, and fallopian tubes. This can lead to scarring and inflammation. Pelvic pain and infertility are common in women with endometriosis.

- **Polycystic ovary syndrome (PCOS)**—results from too much androgen hormone production, which affects ovulation. Ovaries may not release an egg regularly or may not release a viable, healthy egg. Among women who have PCOS, even when a healthy egg is released and fertilized, the uterus may not be receptive to implantation of a fertilized egg.

- **Ovulation disorders**—occur when disruption in the part of the brain that regulates ovulation causes low levels of luteinizing hormone (LH) and follicle-stimulating hormone (FSH). Even slight irregularities in the hormone system can prevent the ovaries from releasing eggs (anovulation).

- **Elevated prolactin (hyperprolactinemia)**—due to high levels of the hormone prolactin, which stimulates breast milk production. This may affect ovulation in women who aren't pregnant or nursing.

- **Early menopause (premature ovarian failure)**—is defined as the absence of menstruation and the early depletion of ovarian follicles before age 40. Certain conditions are associated with early menopause, including immune system diseases, radiation or chemotherapy treatment, and smoking.

- **Fallopian tube damage or blockage**—usually results from inflammation of the fallopian tube (salpingitis). Tubal damage may result in a pregnancy in which the fertilized egg is unable to make its way through the fallopian tube to implant in the uterus (ectopic pregnancy).

- **Uterine fibroids**—are basically benign tumors in the wall of the uterus, common in women in their thirties and forties. Rarely, they may cause infertility by blocking the fallopian tubes. More often, fibroids interfere with proper implantation of the fertilized egg.

- **Pelvic adhesions**—occur when bands of scar tissue bind organs after pelvic infection, appendicitis, or abdominal or pelvic surgery. This scar tissue formation may impair fertility.

- **Thyroid problems**—includes disorders of the thyroid gland, either too much thyroid hormone (hyperthyroidism) or too little (hypothyroidism), can interrupt the menstrual cycle and cause infertility.

Male Infertility

The male fertility process involves the production of mature sperm that must reach and fertilize the egg. Although it may seem to be a simpler process than female fertility, male fertility also requires many conditions to be met. The male must be able to have and sustain an erection, have enough sperm and semen to carry the sperm to the egg, and have sperm of the right shape that move in the right way. A problem meeting any of these conditions contributes to infertility.[10]

Less medical research has been done in the area of male infertility, partly because doctors will tend to recommend Assisted Reproductive Technology (ART) or insemination (discussed in greater detail in chapter 3) as the solution to male infertility. As a result, there are fewer treatment options to assist the underlying medical conditions of male factor infertility.

Again, though not exhaustive, here are some common causes of male infertility[11]:

Impaired production or function of sperm: Most cases of male infertility are due to problems with the sperm, such as

- **Impaired shape and movement of sperm**—occurs when sperm is unable to reach or penetrate the egg due to abnormal sperm structure (morphology) or impaired sperm mobility (motility).

- **Low sperm concentration**—is indicated by a count of ten million or fewer sperm per milliliter of semen. In many instances, no cause for reduced sperm production is found. When sperm concentration is less than five million per milliliter of semen, genetic causes could be involved.

- **Varicocele**—occurs when a varicose vein in the scrotum that may prevent normal cooling of the testicle, leading to reduced sperm count and motility.

- **Undescended testicle**—occurs when one or both testicles fail to descend from the abdomen into the scrotum during fetal development. Because the testicles are exposed to the higher internal body temperature, sperm production may be affected.

- **Testosterone deficiency (male hypogonadism)**—can result from disorders of the testicles themselves or from an abnormality affecting the hypothalamus or pituitary gland in the brain that produces the hormones that control the testicles.

- **Genetic defects**—include instances like Klinefelter's syndrome, which is when a man has two X chromosomes and one Y chromosome instead of one X and one Y. This causes abnormal development of the testicles, resulting in low or absent sperm production and possibly low testosterone.

- **Infections**—may temporarily affect sperm motility. Repeated bouts of sexually transmitted diseases (STDs), such as chlamydia and gonorrhea, are most often associated with male infertility. These infections can cause scarring and block sperm passage. If mumps, a viral infection usually affecting young children, occurs after puberty, inflammation of the testicles can impair sperm production. Inflammation of the prostate (prostatitis), urethra, or epididymis also may alter sperm motility.

- **Impaired delivery of sperm**—may include sexual issues such as erectile dysfunction, premature ejaculation, painful intercourse (dyspareunia), or psychological or relationship problems; retrograde ejaculation (when semen enters the bladder during ejaculation rather than emerging out through the penis); blockage of epididymis or ejaculatory ducts; no semen (ejaculate) resulting from spinal cord injuries or diseases; anti–sperm antibodies, which weaken or disable sperm; cystic fibrosis, which causes a missing or obstructed vas deferens.

In some cases, health care providers cannot determine a cause for infertility in the man or woman, while some known causes of infertility lack any clear-cut treatments.

Carmen relates the challenges of discovering multiple reasons for their difficulty conceiving and the lack of straight-forward treatment options:

> After a few more months, we did more testing, and my husband, Alex, was tested via semen analysis for the first time. This was the first time we realized there might be something wrong with him and not just me. We were both frustrated at how much time had passed, how we had seemingly wasted time, as well as how the addition of Alex's medical issues complicated the situation. More time elapsed, and after two years, we went to see an ob-gyn who put me on Clomid, which is a prescription drug that assists with fertility. My husband began taking a bunch of supplements, started seeing several urologists, and also was prescribed Clomid as well as antibiotics. After taking all these pills, his test results continued to come back the same. Recently, after more than two and a half years of infertility, Alex underwent surgery to correct a varicocele to see if that would help our chances of conceiving.

Secondary Infertility

Secondary infertility is defined as the inability to become pregnant, or carry a pregnancy to term, following the birth of one or more biological children. Those who suffer from secondary infertility often feel like they are especially alone, as if they do not belong in either the fertile or infertile world. The added pressure of feeling like others may judge you for desiring more children when you already have one or more children is a common source of stress. There are even some who feel that secondary infertility is not "real" infertility.

Carmen shares her experience with secondary infertility after the birth of her two children:

> Secondary infertility begs the question of whether we are forcing God's plan. Are we simply not meant to have chil-dren, or more than what we have? As my friends contin-ued to have more children, I have been told I am "falling behind," and it's hard to hear those types of comments. In addition to having a strong desire or calling to raise more

of God's children, there is the added pressure of children asking for a sibling. Every night without fail, our sweet daughter, Monica, asks for a brother or sister, if it is God's will. Her "faith like a child" is an example to us, and she has the faith I need.

This fear of not being able to give our child a brother or sister is common among those who suffer from secondary infertility. I was never too bothered by the fact that I'm an only child, but I have never wanted the same for my own family. I have to remind myself that just because I think something is best does not mean that is what God thinks. My mother wanted a huge family and only had one child. I also try to remember that there are some very important "onlys" in our faith, starting with Jesus himself and his mother Mary, as well as John the Baptist. All of them played a role in our salvation, and we should not minimize the impact of one child, one life.

How Is Infertility Diagnosed?

Although the inability to achieve a pregnancy within a twelve-month period may be an indication of possible infertility, only a health care provider can provide a diagnosis of infertility. If you suspect you may have infertility issues, we suggest seeing your doctor and expressing your interest in finding the underlying causes of your infertility. As with any disease, it is not enough to simply treat the symptoms of infertility. Doctors should first of all ensure that the couple is timing intercourse correctly. (Natural Family Planning, for example, is one method used to assess optimum fertility in women.)

Tests to diagnose the causes of infertility include (but are not limited to):

- blood work, physical examination, and semen sample for men to determine sperm viability; and
- blood work and assessment of the competence of the uterus, ovaries, and fallopian tubes via imaging techniques.

Angelique explains the process she and her husband underwent to get medical answers as to why they were not conceiving:

> Because of my textbook twenty-eight-day cycles and because we practiced NFP and knew we were timing intercourse correctly, we decided to speak to my gynecologist after about six months of trying to conceive. He analyzed our NFP charts and said everything looked good and that it would likely just be a matter of time. We continued to press him, however, and he agreed to have my husband and me get blood drawn. When these produced results that did not indicate any issues, my husband had a semen analysis and I had a hysterosalpingogram (a special ultrasound in which contrast is injected into the uterus to check if the fallopian tubes are open or blocked). Everything checked out okay with these tests, too. It was frustrating to have the nondiagnosis of "unexplained infertility" and not have recourse to any treatments because there were seemingly no underlying issues.

As we can see from the varied diagnoses and experiences of infertility, no two journeys are quite the same, yet we are united in our quest for medical solutions and spiritual guidance. Prayer can help us along our journey:

St. David's Infertility Prayer

Thank you, Lord, for all the blessings in my life. Help me to remember them as I face the challenges of infertility. I pray that I can surrender myself into your hands. Let me accept the reality of this situation and have the wisdom and courage to take action where I can. Strengthen my body, mind and spirit to endure the trials of infertility. Keep me ever mindful of the needs of others and grant us your peace. Amen.[12]

Further Reading

Hannemann, Jeannie, and Bruce Hannemann. *Infertility Journey: Making Faith-Informed Decisions Under the Guiding Hands of God.* Booklet. Kaukauna, WI: Elizabeth Ministry International, n.d.

Taylor, Jameson, and Jennifer Taylor. "Babies Deserve Better: What You Need to Know If You're Struggling with Infertility." *Catholic Answers.* Accessed September 8, 2011. www.catholic.com/thisrock/2006/0604fea3.asp.

*W*hat Does the Catholic Church Have to Do with Infertility?

Faith is a sounder guide than reason. Reason can only go so far, but faith has no limits.

Blaise Pascal

Angelique's Story

My wedding day was a blur to me, filled with so many wonderful memories that they all blend together into one big, happy event that flew by in an instant; but there is one particular moment during the sacrament that stood out to me: when the priest asked if I would "accept children lovingly from God, and bring them up according to the law of Christ and his Church," I remember knowing that my "I do"

12

would mean a huge responsibility, one that, truth be told, I was a bit fearful to undertake.

But there was one word in that important vow I took that I seemed to have overlooked: *receive*. My husband and I didn't realize the importance of that little word *receive* until we faced month after month of dashed hopes as we tried to *have* our first child. Confronted with the possibility of another word we had never paid any attention to—infertility—we began to realize that children are not ours to have; they are God's to give. We are mere recipients of this gift. Thus began our quest to learn the ins and outs of infertility—and what the Catholic Church has to say about it.

Informing and Forming Our Consciences

Though it may seem like a recent phenomenon, infertility has been around as long as humans have. We can see many examples of this in the Bible, such as Sarah (Gn 16–18, 21) and Elizabeth (Lk 1). Infertility has changed through the years, however. It used to be that there wasn't much an infertile couple could do except pray and maybe try some old wives' tales. Now, technology has given couples a much greater degree of perceived control and power. Advances in science have created an array of temptations to pursue treatments that were not readily available to previous generations. Though advances in technology are generally good, we cannot assume that what is technically possible is always morally right.

This is why it is extremely important to educate ourselves on various infertility treatment options and their moral implications. By doing so, we will be properly forming and informing our consciences, which requires consulting God's wisdom in the form of the scriptures, the catechism, papal instructions, and Church documents. We list many of these documents and passages in this book. We should also pray for God's help to internalize and be obedient to the teachings that most challenge us.

Unfortunately, the word *obedience* has a negative connotation. We may think of our parents scolding us as children or even of possibly training a dog, but we don't think of it as something we want to do ourselves. Yet, as challenging as this is, we are each called to be obedient. It is a crucial part of our relationship as God's creation. Interestingly, the word *obedience* comes from *oboedire*, which includes the root word for "to hear." Obedience simply means hearing or listening.

God doesn't only work through us and what we think. He uses our friends and family as well as the Church to speak to us. The scriptures tell us, "Oh, that today you would hear his voice: Do not harden your hearts" (Ps 95:7–8). We know how hard it can be to see the truth in the Church's teaching. The pain of infertility can be so profound it can cloud our vision and make us only focus on one goal—having a baby. But in the end, "what profit is there for one to gain the whole world and forfeit his life?" (Mk 8:36). With obedience, we can properly hear God's voice as we walk along this infertility journey instead of allowing society to dictate our decisions.

This is particularly challenging when one considers all the competing voices in the world. We must know God well enough to recognize his voice above all others in the stirring of our consciences. God should first be our friend, as Blessed Teresa of Calcutta said. The Lord is our Good Shepherd, and "the sheep follow him, because they recognize his voice. But they will not follow a stranger; they will run away from him, because they do not recognize the voice of strangers" (Jn 10:4–5). When reading Church teaching, we form our consciences and learn to recognize God's loving voice. In a similar way, if we learn to recognize God's voice and his promptings in our everyday life, we will be better equipped to hear his voice while navigating the confusing world of infertility treatments, instead of the voice of the stranger that we do not recognize.

As we continue the process of forming our consciences, we may begin to question some of the treatments that were previously acceptable to us. We have friends who, after pursuing multiple rounds of artificial insemination, began feeling uneasy about their situation and halted treatment. They didn't know why they felt this way at the time because their deeper Catholic formation didn't come until later, but they had a nagging sense that something just wasn't right. In our faith tradition, this instinctual feeling that our actions are wrong is called natural law, which "expresses the original moral sense which enables man to discern by reason the good and the evil, the truth and the lie" (*Catechism of the Catholic Church* [*CCC*], 1954). The truth of natural law is written in our hearts, and as St. Augustine says, our hearts are restless until they rest in God. So, it is likely that, in the instance of our friends who halted treatment, their original feeling of uneasiness was the Holy Spirit tugging on their hearts to make a change.

In addition to the natural law with which we are all imbued, scripture and Church teaching also help guide us in knowing right from wrong. The sixth Beatitude proclaims, "Blessed are the pure in heart, for they shall see God" (Mt 5:8). The *Catechism of the Catholic Church* tells us that "pure in heart" refers to those who have attuned their intellects and wills to the demands of God's holiness, chiefly in three areas: charity; chastity or sexual rectitude; love of truth and ortho-doxy of faith (*CCC* 2518). Thus, we are reminded that purity of heart, of body, and of faith are intimately connected and that the faithful are called to live out these beliefs "so that by believing they may obey God, by obeying may live well, by living well may purify their hearts, and with pure hearts may understand what they believe" (*CCC* 2518).

This teaching reminds us that the Church is for us, not against us, when it comes to helping us walk this arduous path of infertility. The Church is our mother, and just as the loving parents we also desire to be, it seeks only our good. We need only open our minds and our hearts to understanding why it teaches as it does. Angelique explains her initial encounter with Church teaching on infertility treatment:

> I had always heard that the Church did not accept some infertility treatments, but before we were faced with infertility, I never knew why. I am an avid researcher by nature and as the months continued to pass without a

positive pregnancy test, I began doing online searches on the Catholic Church and infertility. I don't know what surprised me most about what I found: the wealth of Church materials on the subject or the fact that the information is not widely known. Initially, what I read overwhelmed me because of how profound it was; later, as I continued to read it and pray about it, that same material overwhelmed me because it made me realize God's profound love for me.

Imago Dei

It is with this profound love that God created each of us. "God created man in his image; in the divine image he created him; male and female he created them" (Gn 1:27). Human life is therefore sacred, and the Church speaks out of love in defense of human dignity. We are different from the rest of God's creation, and the creation story in Genesis reminds us of this truth. Every human life, from the moment of conception until death, is sacred because the human person has been willed for its own sake in the image and likeness of the living and holy God (*CCC* 2319). It makes sense then that the propagation of humans would also be special.

St. Ignatius of Loyola begins his seminal Spiritual Exercises with what he calls the Principle and Foundation. This is the starting point of the Exercises because, in order to make wise decisions and follow Christ, St. Ignatius felt we first needed to have the appropriate vision of our purpose. Like Genesis, the Principle and Foundation points to being created in God's image.

Spiritual Exercise 23

Human beings are created to praise, reverence, and serve God our Lord, and by this means embrace salvation. The other things on the face of the earth are created for us, to help us attain the end for which we are created. Therefore, we should use these other things insofar as they help us attain this goal, and turn away from these other things insofar as they impede us from attaining this goal.

As long as we are allowed free choice, we must make ourselves indifferent to all created things. Consequently, as far as we are concerned, we should not prefer health to sickness, riches to poverty, honor to dishonor, a long life to a short life. The same holds for all other things. Our one desire and choice should be that which leads us to the end for which we are created.

The Principle and Foundation can be studied in great detail and meditated upon for hours, but let's focus on the first sentence: "Human beings are created . . . ." St. Ignatius wants to emphasize our creaturehood and, as such, remind us of the fact that we are not God, despite our desire to become like God (Gn 2:16–17). Because we are not God, we cannot create on our own accord. So when we conceive a child, we co-create with God and could not do so by any other means. "In [God's] hand is the life of every living thing and the breath of all mankind" (Jb 12:10).

Endowed with Dignity

Though we are not gods, we are endowed with God-given dignity. A human embryo is conferred all the dignity given to creatures made in the image and likeness of God (*CCC* 2274). As such, our bodies are extremely important, and God's incarnation reveals this to us, as Jesus was the Word made flesh, completely human and completely divine. Because of the Incarnation, our bodies have taken on a special role. "Through the fact that the Word of God became flesh, the body entered theology . . . through the main door" (Tb 23:4). We need to understand that our spirituality is incarnational in that it is lived in and through our bodies; hence, what we do with our bodies is of utmost importance. The Church places such incredible value on each human being, which is why it defends so strongly its right care, from conception until natural death.

The Vatican's 1995 *Charter for Health Care Workers* reiterates the same teaching:

> The body cannot be treated as a belonging. It cannot be dealt with as a thing or an object of which one is the owner and arbiter. Every abusive intervention on the body is an insult to the dignity of the person and thus to God who is its only and absolute Lord: "The human being is not master of his own life: he receives it in order to use it, he is not the proprietor but the administrator, because God alone is Lord of life." (*Charter for Health Care Workers*, 42)

John Paul II's Theology of the Body tells us that, as Lord of life, God has imbued the human body with His "language" of love: "I am yours, and you are mine." This call to communion with Him is the deepest meaning of masculinity and femininity. This language has four characteristics: free, total, faithful, and fruitful. When any one of these four characteristics of marital love is missing in our relationships, we "speak" against love; we are using. We should never treat the body as a thing—as something we own and are free to use as we wish. Instead, we should recognize the body as being made to enflesh God's image and likeness and called to express a love that is free, total, faithful, and fruitful.

Procreative and Unitive

A common societal misconception is that the Catholic Church doesn't desire our sexual relations in marriage to be enjoyable—that it views children as the only end of sex. This couldn't be further from the truth. The Church proclaims God's design for our sexual intimacy to be *both* unitive (uniting the spouses in mutual self-giving love) and procreative (open to the creation of life).

The Church speaks boldly about the dangers of artificially separating these truths of married sexual love. The catechism states that "the spouses' union achieves the twofold end of marriage: the good of the spouses themselves and the transmission of life. These two meanings or values of marriage cannot be separated without altering the couple's spiritual life and compromising the goods of marriage and the future of the family" (*CCC* 2363). Thus there are two potential dangers that may arise from separating these two meanings: either a preoccupation with the procreative element of sex (desiring a baby over all else at the expense of the unitive aspect) or a contraceptive mentality that values the unitive, pleasurable aspect of sex over the creation of new life.

As Catholics, we are called to be countercultural and combat the societal view that separates the procreative and unitive aspects of our sexuality. Perhaps part of society's diminished value of sex can be pinpointed precisely to this divorce of sex's two purposes. Blessed John Paul II reiterated this: "The two dimensions of conjugal union, the unitive and the procreative, cannot be artificially separated without damaging the deepest truth of the conjugal act itself."[1]

The Problem of Infertility

We have both been involved in archdiocesan marriage preparation retreats with our husbands since shortly after we were married (ten years for Carmen and Alex; eight years for Angelique and Richard), and through these programs we are reminded of the importance of the unitive and procreative components of marital love. Due to this knowledge, it is difficult when our sexual relations do not result in children; it is hard not to feel that this is a missing element of our conjugal love. The key to remember is intention and the meaning of the sexual act: as long as we do not act against procreation, we are allowing our marital embrace to renew our wedding vows, uniting us in one flesh, while also remaining open to God's creative power within us. We can't control the outcome, but we can certainly control the intention.

It's encouraging to know that, despite the outcome of our relations, these inseparable unitive and procreative aspects of marital love mirror God's love for us: God loves us so much that he desires to be closer to us, to be one with us (unitive), and so he sent his only begotten son, Jesus, to give us new life (procreative). In other words, God isn't asking us to do anything he hasn't already done himself.

But just because he has already given us his example of unitive and procreative love does not mean that emulating that self-giving love in our own lives is easy. These concepts of love, sex, and our bodies challenged us to acquire a whole new perspective, especially in light of infertility. Accepting the Church's teachings on sex and procreation is challenging because mainstream society offers us very different, often enticing opposing views. It is easy to fall into the trap of listening to what others say the Church teaches instead of going to the source itself. One couple we know shared how they regret not going to the catechism for answers when they were faced with infertility, but they admit they were afraid of what the Church might teach on the matter.

Embracing the Church's stance has been freeing and healing for us. Thanks to these teachings that have helped us to realize our dignity and accept our worth before God, we are impelled to make choices that befit our dignity and worth. Prayer and ongoing reflection on the issues has enabled us to grow to love the Church's teachings both on human dignity and on reproductive technologies (described in chapter 3).

Forks in the Road

Sometimes the issue is not coming to terms with Church teaching but realizing that God's plan for us may not include bearing children. This is especially real for couples that feel their biological clock is ticking. As the years pass, it can be difficult to not begin to wonder if it is too late to have biological children. Though fertility does dramatically decline with age, God's timing for the end of our childbearing years is menopause. Until that point, all things are possible with God, as we remember in the Magnificat. Elizabeth was supposedly too old and yet she is the mother of Jesus' cousin, John the Baptist. St. Anne is someone else we can look to in this situation, as she became the mother of Mary at an advanced age.

There are tests that can be done to check on ovarian reserve and give a better indication of future fertility. It is important to find peace regardless of the situation; through prayer and constant contact with God we can find peace in the choice. There are also increased risks to both mother and child as the mother's age increases. Discernment is very important—God may be calling you to adoption, for example, or perhaps to live a child-free life.

The catechism states that "spouses to whom God has not granted children can nevertheless have a conjugal life full of meaning, in both human and Christian terms. Their marriage can radiate a fruitfulness of charity, of hospitality, and of sacrifice" (*CCC* 1654). We know a middle-aged couple in our community that has done just this. Though child free, they have led fruitful lives in the Church, she by helping homeless mothers find jobs and homes; he by serving in music and Catholic radio ministry.

Getting to the point of making this decision does involve a process of grieving. There is an important distinction to be made between childless and child free. Child free means not having your own children, whereas childless implies not having children in your life. You can then choose to use your maternal and paternal instincts in new ways: perhaps becoming involved in the lives of nieces, nephews, or godchildren; or helping needy children in the community, such as through an organization like Big Brothers, Big Sisters. If dealing with children is too difficult, perhaps helping the elderly will fulfill the nurturing desire you have. It is a process to realize that perhaps our vision of family is not what God had in mind.

It can also be helpful to ask for Mary's intercession since she understands what it is like to obey and trust God without fully understanding. The Lord can also help us understand and assimilate our Church's teachings on the meaning and purpose of sexuality.

Prayer for Purity of Heart

L ord, help me to accept and receive my sexuality as a gift
  from you. Grant me the grace to resist the many lies that
distort this divine gift and help me to live my sexuality according to the truth of self-giving love. Grant me purity of heart so
that I might see the image of your glory in the beauty of others, and one day see you face to face. Amen.[2]

Further Reading

John Paul II. "General Audiences: John Paul II's Theology of the
    Body." Eternal Word Television Network. Accessed September
    12, 2011. www.ewtn.com/library/papaldoc/jp2tbind.htm.

Theology of the Body Institute. Home page. Accessed September
    12, 2011. www.tobinstitute.org/default.asp.

West, Christopher. Home page. Accessed September 12, 2011.
    www.christopherwest.com/default.asp.

Chapter 3

Reproductive Technology and the Catholic Church

The Christian ideal has not been tried and found wanting.
It has been found difficult and left untried.

G. K. Chesterton

It is one thing to agree with a particular rule when one is not faced with the temptation to break it, but once the situation is real rather than merely theoretical, boundaries become barriers between where we are and where we want to be. In the case of infertility, Assisted Reproductive Technology (ART) and its alluring promises of a child become a viable temptation for the couple wrestling with the desperation and many powerful emotions that come with the desire to bear a child. Angelique shares how she handled this reality:

> While experiencing infertility, I often felt like treatments such as insemination or ART were like a carrot being dangled in front of us while we plodded along the seemingly endless road. When we were first beginning tests, my doctor, whom I have known for many years and who knows our beliefs, said something to the effect of "There's always insemination, but I assume you would choose not to do that." My husband and I both said no because we knew the Church was against it (and so did my doctor), but the question that came to mind was "why not?" I know it's important to heed Church teaching, but I wouldn't have been able to articulate at that point why the Church says no. Reading the catechism, scripture, and Church documents helped me to understand that the Church really does have my best interests in mind.

What Is Assisted Reproductive Technology?

The Centers for Disease Control and Prevention (CDC) define Assisted Reproductive Technology as all fertility treatments in which *both* eggs and sperm are extracted. "In general, ART procedures involve surgically removing eggs from a woman's ovaries, combining them with sperm in the laboratory, and returning them to the woman's body or donating them to another woman."[1] ART does not include treatments in which only sperm are extracted and inserted into a woman's uterine cavity (intrauterine insemination) or into the genital tract (artificial insemination) for conception to occur within the woman. ART also does not include procedures in which a woman takes medicine to stimulate egg production without the intention of having eggs retrieved.

The CDC states that ART has been used in the United States since 1981 to help women become pregnant, most commonly through in vitro fertilization (discussed below). According to the CDC's 2008 ART Success Rates Report, 148,055 ART cycles were performed at 436 reporting clinics in the United States during 2008, resulting in 46,326 live births (deliveries of one or more living infants) and a total of 61,426 infants. Although the use of ART is still relatively rare compared to the potential demand, its use has doubled over the past decade. Today, more than 1 percent of all infants born in the United States every year are conceived using ART.[2]

What Does the Church Say About ART and Insemination?

In her wisdom, the Church differentiates between the technologies that honor the dignity of the couple and the life they are to create and those that devalue human life. Our human nature is both corporal and spiritual; therefore, any medical treatment we choose has spiritual ramifications and consequences. Many medical procedures for treating infertility reduce humans to our biological components, to mere procreative processes at the expensive of the unitive bond, but, as discussed in chapter 2, God created us in his image, and this has important implications. First and foremost is that our human love should reflect the unitive and procreative elements of God's love for us.

> Just as the use of contraception might attempt to create a loving union through sex but intentionally excludes the procreative meaning, so many forms of ARTs might attempt to create a new life but intentionally exclude the unitive meaning. Although it happens in different ways, both of these violate the inseparable link between the two meanings of the gift of human sexuality.[3]

How do we know if a treatment upholds human dignity? The United States Conference of Catholic Bishops (USCCB) has developed a helpful rule of thumb with regard to fertility treatments, to help us determine if a treatment upholds the innate dignity of the human person by maintaining the procreative and unitive components of marital love.

- Any procedure which assists marital intercourse in reaching its procreative potential is moral (licit).

- Procedures which add a "third party" into the act of conception, or which substitute a laboratory procedure for intercourse, are not acceptable (illicit).[4]

Our bishops are essentially guiding us to consider any procedure or treatment that assists marital intercourse with both its unitive and procreative functions. The Church stresses the importance of diagnosing and treating the underlying medical issues that may be impeding the couple from conceiving. However, these treatments should never replace intercourse with a third party or laboratory procedure because then the unitive aspect of marital love is absent. "Simply put, life-making and love-making must stay united. The gift of life and the gift of love are inseparable parts of a marital union."[5]

Carmen shares how important it was for her and her husband to be informed on the Church's opinion on these technologies:

> A huge help for us was having friends who had walked the road of infertility ahead of us. As such, we were pretty informed on Church teaching and moral issues before starting the journey ourselves. Once we were faced with the treatment choices, we wanted to understand why the Church teaches what it does, and we read up on the subject. I think it was critical that we understood both what the Church teaches and why it does so. As most people who walk this road, we were offered treatments that we morally objected to, but understanding what these entailed ahead of time and studying Church teaching helped us remain strong in the choices we made.

In this chapter, we will focus on what the Church teaches specifically on insemination and in vitro fertilization. These are not the only reproductive technologies to treat infertility, but they are the most common. Many of the other procedures (detailed in the appendix) are either derived from these procedures or used in conjunction with either of these treatments.

As we delve further into morally and ethically accepted versus unacceptable treatments, it helps to ask ourselves,

- Does this procedure assist the marital act or introduce a third party and replace the marital act?

Insemination: IUI and AID

In our experience and in those of many of our friends, intrauterine insemination (IUI) seems to be the starting point of treatments offered by most mainstream doctors dealing with infertility. IUI is an infertility treatment in which the woman is injected with specially prepared, washed sperm. Sometimes the woman is also treated with medicines that stimulate ovulation before IUI. This procedure is often used to treat mild male factor infertility and couples with unexplained infertility. It is also used with women who have problems with their cervical mucus (if their mucus is a hostile environment for sperm, for example), and the sperm is inserted in her uterine cavity in order to bypass the cervical mucus that may kill the sperm. The sperm used in this procedure may be from either the woman's husband or a donor.

Similar to this treatment is artificial insemination by donor (AID, also called heterologous artificial insemination), which uses the injection of donor sperm that is not from the woman's husband to insert into the woman's genital tract instead of the uterine cavity.

With regard to this procedure, the *Catechism of the Catholic Church* states that "techniques that entail the dissociation of husband and wife by the intrusion of a person other than the couple (donation of sperm or ovum, or surrogate uterus) are gravely immoral. These techniques (heterologous artificial insemination and fertilization) infringe the child's right to be born of a father and mother known to him and bound to each other by marriage" (*CCC* 2376).

The idea that a third party is intimately involved in the physical conception of a child—a technician, a doctor, or a donor—can be very intrusive. The catechism further says that these techniques "betray the spouses' 'right to become a father and mother only through each other'" (*CCC* 2376). In the case of donor gametes (eggs and sperm), this "third-party invasion of the exclusive marriage covenant [is] a kind of mechanical adultery."[6]

In addition to the catechism, other teachings ("Instructions") were developed by the magisterium of the Catholic Church to explain the objections the Church has to some of these technologies. The main teaching of the Church on the subject can be found in the "Instruction on Respect for Human Life in Its Origin and on the Dignity of Creation: Replies to Certain Questions of the Day" (also known as *Donum Vitae* or *DV*). This "Instruction" established that some methods of treating infertility are moral, while others—because they do violence to the dignity of the human person and the institution of marriage—are immoral.

A simple yet essential principle set forth in this document is that the ends do not justify the means. Yes, the end result of a child is wonderful, good, and pure, but how we go about achieving this end is a completely different story. "By comparison with the transmission of other forms of life in the universe, the transmission of human life has a special character of its own, which derives from the special nature of the human person" (*DV* 4). "The child has the right to be conceived, carried in the womb, brought into the world and brought up within marriage" (*DV* II.A.1). In the case of AID, not only is the procedure replacing intercourse, but a third party is also being introduced, both of which go against the USCCB's rule of thumb stated above.

Insemination: AIH

Another related form of insemination is artificial insemination with husband's sperm (AIH), also called homologous artificial insemination, in which the sperm is injected into the genital tract for conception within the woman's body.

While trying to conceive their first child, our friends Andrew and Sarah tried a few months of hormone shots and about four to six rounds of AIH, all of which were unsuccessful.

"We were not walking with the Lord at the time; even though I was aware of him, I ignored him," Sarah explained. "I just knew it wasn't right and yet we just went along. I remember just feeling it was so wrong. In my heart, I felt it was wrong. How desperate we were to have a kid. We felt it was our only option. We were following what the world tells you."

On the subject of AIH, the catechism states that

> techniques involving only the married couple (homologous artificial insemination and fertilization) are perhaps less reprehensible [than those with donors], yet remain morally unacceptable. They dissociate the sexual act from the procreative act. The act which brings the child into existence is no longer an act by which two persons give themselves to one another, but one that "entrusts the life and identity of the embryo into the power of doctors and biologists and establishes the domination of technology over the origin and destiny of the human person." (CCC 2377)

In 2008, another "Instruction" went further than the catechism and *DV* to address some of the new procedures in the area of human reproduction that have arisen since *DV* was written in 1987. The document is entitled "Instruction *Dignitas Personae* on Certain Bioethical Questions" (*DP*), by William Cardinal Levada, prefect of the Congregation for the Doctrine of the Faith.[7]

With regard to artificial insemination by the husband, *DP* states, "Homologous artificial insemination within marriage cannot be admitted except for those cases in which the technical means is not a substitute for the conjugal act, but serves to facilitate and to help so that the act attains its natural purpose."[8] The Church is specifically addressing its concern here over the means used in insemination. Part of what makes insemination illicit is that, in the majority of cases, the sperm is obtained through masturbation.

> The Magisterium of the Church, in the course of a con-
> stant tradition . . . [has] firmly maintained that masturba-
> tion is an intrinsically and gravely disordered action. The
> deliberate use of the sexual faculty, for whatever reason,
> outside of marriage is essentially contrary to its purpose
> . . . [and is] outside of "the sexual relationship which is
> demanded by the moral order and in which the total
> meaning of mutual self-giving and human procreation in
> the context of true love is achieved." (*CCC* 2352)

In other words, masturbation constitutes a grave sin, and
in the case of reproductive treatments, it is not open to life
within the womb. In its "Reproductive Technology Guidelines
for Catholic Couples," the USCCB states that among the reproductive technologies in disagreement with Catholic teachings
are (1) "obtaining a sample of seminal fluid by masturbation"
and (2) "artificial insemination by a non-spouse (AID), or even
by the husband (AIH) if the sample is obtained and handled
by non-licit means (masturbated specimen)."[9]

Masturbation essentially fails to honor the twofold procreative and unitive purposes of the sexual union. The sperm
used in these procedures (which is often immorally obtained
with the aid of pornography to assist the male with achieving
a sperm sample) is usually then prepared and washed, and in
some cases, the best sperm is selected to be injected into the
woman—hence, some of it remains unused.

The Church deems morally licit an alternative means for
collecting sperm (either for the purposes of diagnosing sperm
quality or in the use of licit treatments) that does not interrupt or degrade the marital act. "Seminal fluid samples can
be obtained from a non-lubricated, perforated condom after
normal intercourse."[10]

Therefore, insemination may be licit when the sample is
obtained through normal intercourse with the use of a perforated condom. The issue, though, is that most doctors would
not allow you to collect the specimen in this way as they
would likely prefer to have control over which are the best

sperm to inject into the woman. Additionally, the procedure still introduces a third party by having someone else do the insemination. If you and your spouse are considering AIH with licitly obtained semen, we encourage you to ask the Holy Spirit for guidance and read what the Church has written on the subject to determine what you are being called to do. Chapter 5 on discernment may help you with this decision.

In Vitro Fertilization—IVF

In vitro fertilization (IVF) is when conception occurs outside the body "in a glass" (*in vitro* is Latin for "in glass"). It is now one of the most common approaches for achieving pregnancy when facing infertility. In IVF, the woman is usually treated with hormones to alter her natural cycle and stimulate her ovaries to produce a number of eggs. The eggs, or ova, are extracted with a needle inserted through either the vagina or the abdomen using an ultrasound as a guide. Ova are then joined in a laboratory with a carefully washed specimen of semen to allow fertilization. Prior to implantation in the woman's uterus, embryos are examined in order to select the "best" ones. Usually at least two embryos are implanted and sometimes more with the hope of getting at least one live baby. Overall success rates in terms of having a living child using IVF range from 16 to 20 percent.[11]

As we have seen, the Church teaches that medical techniques may only assist the procreative act and not replace or substitute it. "Conception should take place within the body, and not outside. A corresponding rule governs the treatment of human embryos [fertilized eggs], who ought to be conceived through the marital act of a loving couple, and not engendered in vitro by a laboratory technician."[12]

The very nature of the procedure goes against God's design for bringing children into the world. Instead of husband and wife coming together in a physical expression of love for one another, a doctor or lab technician acts as a third party that joins the sperm and egg to create a new life.

The Church has said that treatments that assist the couple may be permissible, but IVF replaces the marital act altogether. Through in vitro fertilization, a couple can procreate without ever having sexual relations. Christopher West, a renowned theologian and speaker on Pope John Paul II's Theology of the Body, often says that we have all come into existence because our parents had sex, but this fundamental truth is no longer so. IVF is essentially the flip side of contraception: Rather than trying to have sex without babies, we try to have babies without sex.

West also says human beings can assume two postures in life: receptivity or grasping.[13] He explains that the choice depends on one's concept of God. If we view God as a god who loves us and desires our ultimate happiness, then we place ourselves in a receptive mode. Imagine a person who has both hands open and outstretched, receptive to God's gifts. On the other hand, if we view God as a tyrant who does not want our happiness, then we try to grasp life for ourselves. Visualize a person grasping at something she or he desires with closed fists, closed to what God desires to place there, and instead grabbing at it for themselves. West explains how couples must never shift from receptivity to grasping, and he identifies in vitro fertilization as a form of grasping: "Consciously or unconsciously, those who resort to in-vitro fertilization demonstrate that they are not content with remaining receptive before the One who alone is 'Lord and Giver of life.' Since the Creator has not granted the gift [of a child] through their own self-giving, they seek to 'extort the gift.'"[14]

Children Are a Gift

The concern with procedures like IVF is that the child is viewed as a commercial product instead of a gift from God. "In IVF, children are engendered through a technical process, subjected to 'quality control,' and eliminated if found 'defective.'"[15]

If we who want to be parents view the child as something we can produce on our own, then we are exercising a dominion that God did not intend over another human life. The catechism states that

> such a relationship of domination is in itself contrary to the dignity and equality that must be common to parents and children. Under the moral aspect procreation is deprived of its proper perfection when it is not willed as the fruit of the conjugal act, that is to say, of the specific act of the spouses' union. . . . Only respect for the link between the meanings of the conjugal act and respect for the unity of the human being make possible procreation in conformity with the dignity of the person. (*CCC* 2377)

DP also reminds us that husband and wife cooperate with God in the creation of a new person—they are not givers of life as those who experience infertility know so deeply. Couples need God to transmit that breath of life and create a new human being. Genesis 4:1 says it so well: "I have conceived a child with the help of the Lord." Thus, we are called to conceive with the help of the Lord, not on our own or by taking matters into our own hands. If there is to be any "third party" involved in conception, it is God. The act through which God intended human life to be transmitted involves mutual self-gift, which is not present in some of the medical treatments available. This gift of self can only occur in a personal encounter, not through the use of catheters and petri dishes. "Each child is equal in dignity to his or her mother. This is why the desire for a child, albeit a very real and natural desire, can never become a right to a child at any cost. No person can claim the right to the existence of another; otherwise the latter would be placed on a lower level of value than the one who claims such a right."[16]

We must also consider the feelings of the children who are born of an IVF procedure. They may come to view themselves as a product of our technology, even as a consumer good that their parents have paid for and have a "right" to expect—not as fellow persons who are equal in dignity to their parents. Though the means used to achieve a pregnancy may be illicit, the child is a child of God with all the dignity afforded to all creatures in God's image and likeness. "Human embryos obtained *in vitro* are human beings and subjects with rights: their dignity and right to life must be respected from the first moment of their existence" (*DV* I.5).

The respect that should be shown to a human embryo begins with viewing a child as a gift. "A child is not something *owed* to one, but is a *gift*. The "supreme gift of marriage" is a human person. A child may not be considered a piece of property, an idea to which an alleged "right to a child" would lead. In this area, the child is not the one who possesses genuine rights: the "right to be the fruit of the specific act of the conjugal love of his parents" and "the right to be respected as a person from the moment of his conception" (*CCC* 2378).

Other Moral Concerns of IVF

One of the additional moral concerns with IVF that is addressed in *DP* is the frozen embryos that are created. Because the endometrium is considerably changed by the stimulation of ovaries to produce eggs prior to an IVF procedure, it is the practice in some centers to freeze the embryos and to implant them in a subsequent menstrual cycle. Additionally, due to the superovulation medications that are administered to stimulate the ovaries, numerous ova are extracted for use in the in vitro process. In most instances, multiple embryos are created and only a few are implanted; the rest are frozen.

A quick online search will garner descriptions of the process of freezing embryos (human embryo cryopreservation), which entails creating embryos in a petri dish in order to be frozen and stored. Here is one description found online:

> Techniques of controlled-rate freezing are utilized that slowly cool embryos in cryoprotectant fluid ("anti-freeze" solution) from body temperature down to −196°C, at which temperature they are stored in containers of liquid nitrogen called dewars. The embryos are actually

contained within special indelibly labeled plastic vials, or straws, that are sealed prior to freezing. Once frozen, they are placed inside labeled tubes attached to aluminum cans and stored in numbered canisters within the liquid nitrogen dewar.

When it comes time to thaw the embryos, all available identifiers of the stored specimen must match and be confirmed before thawing commences. The embryos are thawed out at room temperature, which takes about one to two minutes. However, the most critical element of the thaw procedure is not the timing but the careful dilution of the cryoprotectant fluid to return the embryo to its favored culture medium. This permits resumed growth and development in vitro. Once this is done, the embryo is assessed for cryodamage to determine if it is suitable for transfer. Experience has shown that if the embryo survives 50 percent or more intact, it is worthwhile to replace it. Embryos can accommodate such levels of cellular damage and still establish healthy pregnancies. All thawed embryos routinely undergo assisted hatching prior to transfer. The zona pellucida, which surrounds the embryo, has been shown to suffer a certain amount of hardening during cryopreservation. This can be overcome by artificially making an opening in the outer embryo shell.[17]

The description goes on to state that "it is very likely that freezing will cause loss of some embryos, perhaps as many as 25–50 percent of those cryostored." This process seems to completely undermine the fact that we're talking about a child, and not a process by which we're freeze-drying food, for example. This is underscored by the term "frosties," which is often used as a nickname for frozen embryos. In this light, IVF seems like a detached, cold procedure (no pun intended) that fails to uphold the dignity of these human lives.

Many of these frozen embryos are abandoned and never used by couples. Some couples struggle with their preserved embryos and even pay monthly fees to keep them frozen.

The so-called spare embryos may be preserved for future use, donated to other couples or to researchers, or destroyed. Sadly, there are no known statistics on just how many embryos are left unclaimed worldwide, nor for how long.

A woman at our church shared that she had five embryos frozen and she did not know what to do with them. This is a challenging ethical dilemma when one considers the options available to this woman. As Catholics, we believe that life begins at conception and this is true whether life begins in the womb or in a petri dish. As such, these couples have real human lives frozen. Sometimes these embryos are disposed of as if they were a waste product created by IVF. This is tantamount to abortion.

Also, some embryos are often killed during the IVF procedure because the doctors only choose the healthiest one(s) to implant. Others are destroyed. There is also the concern of "selective reduction," which occurs because of the increasing number of embryos that are implanted. Selective reduction is really just a euphemism for abortion. After the embryo has been implanted into the woman's uterus, doctors essentially decide which embryos have the best chance for survival and abort the others to diminish risk to the mother and other embryos that have been implanted. "It does not seem terribly consistent for a treatment program, which is trying to create new life, to end up destroying new life."[18]

In addition to selective reduction, a multiples birth—the birth of more than one child from a single pregnancy, common with IVF due to the hyperovulation medications administered—creates greater risks for the mother and babies. The CDC reports that adverse outcomes have been described both in women undergoing ART and in infants born from these procedures. The risks for mom and baby include but are not limited to ovarian hyperstimulation syndrome, low birth weight, preterm delivery, infant death, and disability among survivors. ART-conceived singletons also face increased risks for low birth weight, preterm delivery, and fetal growth restriction.[19]

As technology evolves, more reproductive procedures are introduced. The Church will have to continue to analyze the advent of these treatments in light of the dignity of the human person.[20]

> The Church offers us a useful road map as we enter this complex territory. New procedures develop daily and details of current ones change frequently, so it is impossible for the Church to list every test, procedure or treatment that the Church does and does not allow. It is better to learn the basis for those decisions. Then you can apply the very fundamental guidelines to each procedure and understand how it can impact your situation.[21]

Cultural Temptations

For most couples experiencing infertility, the first doctor they visit will not necessarily know about or recommend treatments that are in line with Church teaching. The possibility of being offered IVF or IUI by a typical doctor is extremely high, and if a couple's doctor is not invested in helping them make decisions congruent with their faith and personal values, then the couple may find themselves always on the defensive. Or it could become tempting to partake in one of these procedures due to the luring promise that they will be successful. Doctors and science can help infertile couples; it is our job to be cautious with regard to how this help is given. "Applied biology and medicine work together for the integral good of human life when they come to the aid of a person stricken by illness and infirmity and when they respect his or her dignity as a creature of God" (*DV* 3).

We have discovered when speaking to friends who experienced infertility and used ART or insemination that many did not know the treatments they used were immoral. Some admit to not doing research as they should have, and some admit to not really wanting to know. This may also be the case for well-meaning people—doctors, friends, and family members— who may be pushing for some of these treatments as options. By informing ourselves, we can educate them as well.

Angelique summarizes what she discovered when she read what the Church teaches on treating infertility:

> What I found in my own research of Church teachings were two major desires that the Church has for me with regard to infertility: that I care for my body and that I care for my soul. First, the Church desires for me to be as healthy as possible in order to honor the body that God gave me. If I have symptoms of infertility, for example, the Church encourages me to get to the bottom of why this is happening, be it physiological, hormonal, or just a matter of timing. It was encouraging for me to see that if I have a hormonal imbalance, the Church backs taking the appropriate hormones to regulate this imbalance; if I have some sort of physiological condition (blocked fallopian tubes, let's say), then the Church also supports having surgery or other appropriate procedure to fix this. If it's a matter of not timing intercourse properly, then the Church even offers classes in Natural Family Planning to help me realize my optimum fertility. The Church gets a bad rap with regard to accepting modern medical technology, but it really surprised me that the Church was ahead of the game in terms of wanting us to avail ourselves of technology as long as it truly helps to heal us.
>
> The second theme I found is the Church's desire to guard my soul and uphold my God-given dignity. Because the Church knows that some of these treatments do not honor both the procreative and unitive elements of marital love as God designed it, the Church, as my loving mother, says, "No, that's not good for you." She fears that by taking conception into my own hands, I may lose sight of God being my loving Father who ultimately knows what's best for me. Additionally, I am failing to respect my own dignity, my husband's dignity, and my future child's dignity if I begin to manipulate the act of creation and forget that I am a mere co-creator with God. It can be hard to heed the teachings of my mother Church and my Father's Word, but I know from personal experience that not trusting in my parents can have negative ramifications.

This book is not a treatise on the bioethics of some of these issues, so we have included an extensive, but not exhaustive, list of resources at the end of chapters 3 and 4 and in the appendix so that you can become more informed on the subject and truly understand why the Church teaches what it does. The Church is always teaching us like a gentle parent, and it has an obligation to help us form our consciences by teaching the truth.

A final challenge comes from Blessed John Henry Cardinal Newman, who wrote these words to medical students in 1852:

> Trust the Church of God implicitly even when your natural judgment would take a different course from hers and would induce you to question her prudence or correctness. Recollect what a hard task she has; and how she is sure to be criticized and spoken against, whatever she does; recollect how much she needs your loyal and tender devotion; recollect too, how long is the experience gained over so many centuries; and what a right she has to claim your assent to principles which have had so extended and triumphant a trial. Thank her that she has kept the faith safe for so many generations and do your part in helping her to transmit it to generations after you.[22]

Trusting in God and his Church can be challenging in the face of so many competing options. He desires to help us as we choose to follow him—we only need to ask:

Prayer in the Face of Fertility Challenges

Lord, help me to know that You are enough. Take my eyes off of myself. Take my eyes off of the child I desire. Help me to delight myself in You. Mold the desires of my heart to be in line with Your will. I don't want to need to be a mother more than I need to be your humble, obedient child. I don't want wanting to have a baby to be a stumbling block between You and me anymore.

Lord, I want to give this desire, this drive, this ache up to You. Help me not to snatch it back as I so often do with the burdens I place in Your hands. Help me to be truly content with Your will and Your timing.

Lord, You know that I still desire a baby—someone to mold, teach, train, shape, guide, and help to grow in You. But until the day You give me that joyous blessing, help me to grow in You. Let me reach out to those around me. Let me witness and minister to the children You place in my path.

Thank you for lifting my burden. Help me to keep you first! Let me seek Your face daily, and let me know that You are enough![23]

Other Reproductive Treatments

In addition to IVF and IUI using illicitly obtained sperm, the Church has also deemed immoral the following treatments due to the fact that fertilization takes place outside of the womb and third parties are introduced.

- Zygote intrafallopian transfer (ZIFT), in which eggs and sperm are combined as in IVF, but the embryos are immediately transferred to the woman's fallopian tubes without first being examined in a petri dish. Also known as pronuclear stage transfer (PROST).

- Intracytoplasmic sperm injection (ICSI), an addendum to IVF in which eggs and sperm are collected as in IVF but a single sperm is injected into a single egg. The resulting embryo grows in the lab until it reaches the eight- to sixteen- cell stage and then is implanted in the uterus.

- Surrogacy is when an embryo is surgically implanted into a woman's uterus. The woman is either genetically a stranger to the embryo or has contributed the donation of her own ovum, fertilized through insemination with the sperm of a man other than her husband. She carries the pregnancy with a pledge to surrender the baby once it is born.

- Egg/sperm donors, wherein, if there is an issue with a woman's eggs, people will use egg donors to help conceive. Similarly, if a man's sperm is found to be the cause of infertility, sperm donors are used. The problem with donors is the same as with surrogates—they introduce third parties into the equation. Donors deprive the child of the right to be born of its parents. It can even be seen as infidelity to some extent by bringing a third party into the marriage.

The Church has not yet definitively ruled on the following procedures:

- Gamete intrafallopian transfer (GIFT), in which the woman's ovaries are hyperstimulated and the eggs are retrieved, after which they are placed in a catheter with sperm with an air bubble separating the sperm and egg. The catheter is then inserted into the woman's body so that the fertilization can take place within the woman's body.

- Embryo adoption[24] refers to having an abandoned embryo transferred to the uterus of a woman willing to gestate this child to save his or her life. Many have asked whether this might be a legitimate way for conscientious couples to respond, in a potentially life-affirming way, to the problem of thousands of abandoned embryos (also called snowflake children) at IVF clinics in the United States.[25] *Dignitas Personae* makes mention of "prenatal adoption" but does not definitively rule on the subject.[26]

As the number of frozen embryos grows—many of which may never be used—many Catholics may find embryo adoption alluring. Many ethicists debate the morality of embryo adoption, and this book is not meant to be a treatise on the ethical implications of this issue; however, it is very important for us as Catholics to be informed. Part of the debate among ethicists regarding this situation is that the starting point—IVF—is one that is unnatural and that the Church has clearly spoken against. However, the debate centers mostly around what, then, can be done to help these embryos that already exist.

Further Reading

Church Documents

Catechism of the Catholic Church. Nn. 2373–79. Liguori, MO: Liguori, 1994.

Ratzinger, Joseph Cardinal. "Instruction *Donum Vitae*: Instruction on Respect for Human Life in Its Origin and on the Dignity of Procreation. Congregation for the Doctrine of the Faith. February 22, 1987. www.vatican .va/roman_curia/congregations/cfaith/documents/ rc_con_cfaith_doc_19870222_respect-for-human-life_en.html.

Levada, William Cardinal. "Instruction *Dignitas Personae* on Certain Bioethical Questions." Congregation for the Doctrine of the Faith, September 8, 2008. www.vatican .va/roman_curia/congregations/cfaith/documents/ rc_con_cfaith_doc_20081208_dignitas-personae_en.html.

National Catholic Bioethics Center. Home page. Accessed September 15, 2011. www.ncbcenter.org/page.aspx?pid = 183.

Pope John Paul II. "Encyclical *Evangelium Vitae*: On the Value and Inviolability of Human Life." March 25, 1995. www .vatican.va/holy_father/john_paul_ii/encyclicals/ documents/hf_jp-ii_enc_25031995_evangelium-vitae_en.html.

Statements of the Bishops of the United States

United States Conference of Catholic Bishops. *Ethical and Religious Directives for Catholic Health Care Services*. 4th ed. Washington, DC: Author, 2001. See part 4, "Issues in Care for the Beginning of Life," introduction and directives, 38–43.

—— "Life-Giving Love in an Age of Technology." 2009. www .usccb.org/upload/lifegiving-love-age-technology-2009.pdf.

—— "Married Love and the Gift of Life." Washington, DC: USCCB 2006.

—— "On Embryonic Stem Cell Research." Washington, DC: USCCB 2008.

Articles from the Respect Life Program of the Bishops of the United States

Anderson, Marie, and John Bruchalski. "Assisted Reproductive Technologies Are Anti-Woman." Respect Life Program, 2004. http://old.usccb.org/prolife/programs/rlp/04anderson.shtml.

Haas, John M. "Begotten Not Made: A Catholic View of Reproductive Technology." 1998. http://old.usccb.org/prolife/programs/rlp/98rlphaa.shtml.

Klaus, Hanna. "Reproductive Technology (Evaluation and Treatment of Infertility) Guidelines for Catholic Couples." United States Conference of Catholic Bishops, 2009. http://old.usccb.org/prolife/issues/nfp/treatment.shtml.

Mindling, J. Daniel. "Addressing Infertility with Compassion and Clarity." Respect Life Program, 2009. http://old.usccb.org/prolife/programs/rlp/2009/mindlingpamphlet.pdf.

Other Articles

Drake, Tim. "What's Wrong with In-Vitro Fertilization." 2004. www.staycatholic.com/what_is_wrong_with_in-vitro_fertilization.htm.

Incandela, Joseph M. "Catholic Social Thought: Reproductive Technologies." Last updated September 13, 2011. www.saintmarys.edu/~incandel/cst.html#REPRO.

May, William E. "Begetting vs. Making Babies." November 14, 2004. www.christendom-awake.org/pages/may/begetting.htm.

McCarthy, Donald G., ed. *Reproductive Technologies, Marriage and the Church.* Braintree, MA: Pope John XXIII Medical-Moral Research and Education Center, 1988.

Sparks, Richard C. "Helping Childless Couples Conceive." *St. Anthony Messenger.* Accessed September 15, 2011. www.americancatholic.org/Messenger/Apr1997/feature1.asp.

Sweeney, Kathleen Curran. "The Child: Begotten, Not Manmade: Catholic Teaching on In-Vitro Fertilization." 2008. www.kofc .org/un/en/resources/cis/cis330.pdf.

$\mathcal{T}$reatment
Options
for Catholics

The extreme greatness of Christianity lies in the fact that
it does not seek a supernatural remedy for suffering but
a supernatural use for it.

Simone Weil

In an explanation of John Paul II's Theology of the Body
used in a Natural Family Planning (NFP) course taught by
the Couple to Couple League, Father Richard Hogan explains
that it sometimes seems as if the Church is always saying no.
This appears especially true regarding her teaching on sexuality and morality, but in reality the Church is saying yes to a
way of thinking that is different from the rest of society. The
Church says yes to the mystery that we are called to love as
God loves—that, as human beings, we are worthy of a love

greater than that offered by the world and that our choices should reflect this worth we have in God.

This idea that the Catholic Church is always saying no may lead people to believe the Church does not accept any treatment for infertility, but this is far from the truth. The Church's position on accepted treatments essentially addresses the medical conditions that underlie infertility while always acknowledging the intrinsic value of human life. In other words, instead of a quick-fix procedure to achieve pregnancy that sometimes has immoral ramifications, the Church, in her wisdom, desires to heal whatever is not functioning properly in our bodies that may be causing infertility.

In fact, the Church actually sanctions more treatments than it rejects. It's important to recall the United States Conference of Catholic Bishops' "rule of thumb" with regard to fertility treatments (explained in chapter 3): "In a nutshell anything that helps marital intercourse to be more effective is moral; anything that inserts a third party into the act of conception or replaces intercourse is not."[1]

Catholic Solutions

It was precisely with this desire to honor the dual purposes of marital love while also diagnosing the underlying reasons behind infertility that the Pope Paul VI Institute for the Study of Human Reproduction began researching and developing fertility evaluation and treatments that honor marital integrity and respect life. This "Fertility*Care*" system is called Natural Procreative Technology (NaProTECHNOLOGY), and it begins with the premise that infertility may be a result of disorders that disrupt normal ovarian and uterine function. Because these disorders can interfere with conceiving and sustaining a pregnancy, treatments are administered that help alleviate these underlying causes of infertility.

> Many couples have not been exposed to the possibility that reproductive health care can be provided with great efficiency and a high rate of success, while at the

same time being totally and completely consistent with
the beliefs of their Catholic faith. Your doctor or pastor
[to whom you may go for advice] may not yet be aware
of these new developments because, unlike the various
assisted reproductive technologies, very few resources are
available to promote them.[2]

Though NaProTECHNOLOGY started in Omaha,Nebraska,
in the 1960s, Fertility*Care* physicians trained by the Pope Paul
VI Institute to help women's reproductive health are now
found all over the nation. Additionally, Catholic physicians
around the United States have also begun treating infertility patients in accordance with Church teaching in a similar
fashion. "Research aimed at reducing human sterility is to be
encouraged, on condition that it is placed 'at the service of
the human person, of his inalienable rights, and his true and
integral good according to the design and will of God'" (*CCC*
2375). These Catholic physicians who have committed themselves to treating infertility in a comprehensive, moral way
are answering this call to research alternate means of healing
infertility that honor our human dignity.

In *Women, Sex, and the Church,* Katie Elrod wrote a chapter
titled "The Church's Best Kept Secret: Church Teaching on
Infertility Treatment" in which she said,

> For many, the Catholic Church may be the last place they
> thought they would discover such a treasure; for me, it
> confirmed my understanding of the fundamental symbio-
> sis between faith and science. When reproductive technol-
> ogy allows itself to be ordered by respect for the human
> person, it discovers avenues for inquiry that not only pro-
> duce results, but are also in accord with human dignity.[3]

Finding Medical Support

The first step when dealing with medical infertility
options is to familiarize yourself with the treatments that are
accepted by the Church so that you are not persuaded into
pursuing immoral treatments. These can be found at the end

of chapter 3. You can also find a list of ethicists and infertility terms you should know in the appendix to help you be informed. When you are at your doctor's visit, take notes and always ask why something is being prescribed. Sometimes doctors can seem intimidating, and you may feel like you are imposing on their schedules by asking questions. However, in the American health care system patients are customers, and we have a right to understand what we are purchasing when a treatment, test, or prescription is advised. It also helps to have as much information as possible on hand when you visit your doctor. This will make it easier for him or her to assist you in taking the next step rather than ordering a slew of tests and starting from scratch every time. Your physician is also more likely to share more sophisticated insights with you if you demonstrate your understanding of infertility.[4]

It helps to remember that doctors are consultants; they offer recommendations. Physicians work for you, though it may feel differently at times. Treatment decisions are up to you as a couple. When looking for a doctor, try to find someone who meets your needs as a patient and as a person, as this relationship is very important. You should feel comfortable asking questions about your treatment. The doctor, in turn, should be forthcoming with information and explanations. He or she should be willing to answer your questions and concerns. When it comes to making a medical decision, trust your instincts.

These pieces of advice would have been very helpful to me when I was at the beginning of my journey, when a doctor with whom I never felt comfortable was recommended to me. I wanted to like him more than I did, and I tried to for several months, but things were just not right. My questions went unanswered; phone calls were not returned—I seemed to be in a never-ending queue. Seeing the doctor was even more difficult; it reminded me of the *Wizard of Oz* and how you could never see the Wizard himself. Appointments were months and months down the road, which may have been fine had the staff members been available in the interim, but they were not. I knew I needed to switch to another doctor, but I was

afraid of switching because I heard so many success stories
from this highly recommended doctor, and I wanted to be one
of those success stories, too. I did not value the importance of
having a doctor with whom I had a good relationship until I
found a doctor who was a better fit for me. I had to learn that
just because someone else has a wonderful experience with
a particular doctor doesn't guarantee that I will.

I also learned that a gynecologist cannot necessarily treat
infertility in every instance. It may be necessary to see a
reproductive endocrinolo-
gist or an ob-gyn that specializes in Catholic treatment,
depending on the diagnosis.
I am blessed with a wonderful, kind-hearted gynecologist
whom I have been with for
many years, but we reached
a point where there was noth-
ing else he could do for me. He gave me the names of several
specialists he thought might be able to help us. His example
taught me that a good doctor should be comfortable with and
encourage his patients to seek other opinions when necessary.

Questions to ask the practice to help you
become an educated patient:

- How many doctors are in the group?

- What is the role of the nurses?

- If I have a question, who will I speak to?

- What other support staff is available?

The number of doctors in the group can affect the type of
care you receive and how long you wait to see a doctor. For
instance, if there are several doctors in the practice, it may be
easier to get an appointment as long as you are willing to be
seen by any of the doctors in the group. It can also be helpful
if some of the doctors have different specialties, for example,
a surgeon who can perform laparoscopies and a reproductive
endocrinologist who can help with hormone imbalances.

The nurses are the people you will likely speak to the
most, so it is important to understand their roles upfront
and make sure you are comfortable with that. For example,
some patients are fine with communicating with nurses and
having them be intermediaries between the patient and the
physician, but other patients prefer to speak to the physician
directly.

Poor communication, unreturned phone calls, and unanswered questions are all red flags that the practice and its practitioners may be inattentive to your needs. Before you see your doctor you should also research the basic tests that will be run to diagnose infertility, and don't be afraid to ask questions if you don't understand something.

At a point in our journey when we were seeking answers, a doctor ordered a battery of tests, one of which required surgery. I asked for an explanation as to why this was necessary and never received a satisfactory answer. I consulted other doctors, and three of them told me the surgery was unnecessary. The other physicians explained that I had no symptoms that would indicate a need for the surgery, so it would have been exploratory in nature. The surgery would have meant a great deal of financial hardship for my family as well as the risks involved with any surgery. I never had the surgery and instead pursued other treatments that were more conservative and that were specifically designed to treat symptoms and conditions I had.

This experience taught me to avoid letting a doctor or medical practice convince me that they are the only ones who can help me or perform a given procedure. No doctor has a monopoly on healing.

Research different doctors, and if you can find a doctor who shares your values, that can make the process much easier. The website *One More Soul*, which has a wonderful listing of pro-life doctors, is very helpful in finding health care professionals who will respect your beliefs. The American Association of Pro-life Obstetricians and Gynecologists also has a list of pro-life doctors that can be searched by area.[5]

Desperate Times, Drastic Measures

Researching doctors who share our values is important because the despair felt during infertility sometimes tempts us to resort to drastic, unexpected measures.

I live in Miami and am blessed to have wonderful doctors, but there are no Natural Family Planning–only doctors in our area. Because I live in a major metropolitan area, I found it ridiculous to have to travel thousands of miles for treatment, but after an appointment with a local doctor who was not supportive of our beliefs, my perspective changed. I was reminded of how difficult it is to take advice and opinions from someone who you doubt has your best interests in mind. From a financial perspective as well, it can feel like doctors are taking advantage of the desperation that infertile couples experience and that they could charge whatever they want because couples will pay it, banking on the fact that infertile couples would do almost anything for the hope of bearing a child. Ultimately, I decided that traveling thousands of miles to be assured that my entire being is cared for is really a small sacrifice.

St. Ignatius speaks of the importance of "cura personalis," which means the care of the whole person, and it is this holistic approach to medicine that we should be seeking. Unfortunately, some medical doctors are not looking at the patient in a holistic way. They are not considering the body and the spirit. In fact, several doctors—even Catholic doctors—told us that we needed to do intrauterine insemination (IUI) or in vitro fertilization (IVF), but our faith reminds us to consider how that would that damage our souls.

Even though we found more holistic approaches outside of our own city, being treated cross-country wasn't easy. I felt so strange the day I sent my monthly fertility charts across the country for review. And when I look back on it now, my road of infertility seems paved with moments I never thought I would get to. I never thought I would be infertile; I never thought I would reach the three-year mark; and I never thought I would need to send my charts and labs halfway across the country to consult an expert because there are no answers to be found here. But life is full of "I never thought I would . . ." God knows our capabilities and where we should be. He is guiding and accompanying us on the road of infertility.

The Second Letter to the Corinthians 4:17–18 says, "For this momentary light affliction is producing for us an eternal

weight of glory beyond all comparison, as we look not to what
is seen but to what is unseen; for what is seen is transitory,
but what is unseen is eternal."

I certainly do not want to sound negative about doctors
because, though I have been disappointed in some, I have also
been in awe of others. I have an outstanding and compassionate primary care physician who is, more than anything, my
friend. She did research, consulted other doctors, and went
far above the call of duty. She was my advocate when I could
not advocate for myself. And then there were the doctors I
never even met personally but whose pastoral care was healing in more than just a physical way. For example, there was
a doctor whom I never met but who studied my case and was
simply convicted that my infertility was God's way of spacing
our children. Also helpful was another doctor who spoke to
my primary care physician on several occasions and offered
guidance when we did not know how to proceed.

Advocating for Ourselves

One of the most valuable lessons I have learned in my
experience with infertility and the pursuit of answers is that
we must all be our own advocates. I am an attorney, and as
such, I am first and foremost an advocate, a counselor, and an
advisor. For this reason, I have a particular devotion to Our
Lady of Good Counsel and have often sought her intercession
in making decisions, both professionally and personally. She
is a powerful intercessor for anyone trying to discern the best
options on this journey of infertility. As advocates, attorneys
need to research, prepare, and all too often argue a client's
position. We, as patients, have to do the same. I learned not
to blindly take the first doctor's advice I heard but to educate
myself on my options and consult multiple practitioners. It
helps to be prepared with knowledge of which treatments are
licit (see chapter 3) and the best way to talk to your doctor
about prescribing particular treatments.

Additionally, it may be important to advocate for yourself at work as well. In order to have essential tests and be

monitored for treatments it may be necessary to miss work at times. You may need to talk to your supervisor and tell him or her what is happening. We have found that most employers are sympathetic and accommodating of these situations.

Combating Hypochondria

The Internet is an incredible tool and one I certainly do not want to live without. However, the Internet also has the unfortunate ability to make us think we have all sorts of conditions that we probably do not have. In the process of educating ourselves, it helps to keep in mind that not everything we read on the Internet is true or relevant to our own situation. I learned we should have faith and trust in our doctors and avoid thinking we exhibit symptoms for all sorts of conditions. Sometimes reading infertility blogs and seeing the long list of medications and treatments that other couples have gone through, though helpful, may make us think we need to follow the same course of action. However, what is true for one family may not necessarily be the solution for another.

Lifestyle Changes

In our particular situation, we had achieved two pregnancies rather easily and then slowly realized we were not in Kansas anymore. When facing secondary infertility, I remember that my first course of action was to go to Marilyn Shannon's book, *Fertility, Cycles and Nutrition*, and together with my NFP charts, tried to figure out what could be happening and if there was some way to try to improve my cycles with supplements. I realized that I needed to take vitamins to see if it made a difference. I'm sure they helped, but after years of infertility at some point, out of frustration, I stopped taking them. Many months later, I realized that these supplements made me healthier, and whether we achieved a pregnancy or not, I would rather be healthier by taking them.

My husband talks about the frustration of taking dozens of supplements without any guaranteed result. In a similar vein, you may feel like a walking pharmacy, taking pills, injections, and vitamins all day long. Though it can be a challenge, these drugs are intended to help and are key to any successful, natural improvement.

The Couple to Couple League International (CCLI) has seen how diet plays a role in fertility and recommends good, sound nutrition as the first line of defense. Some of the vitamins they recommend are vitamins A and D as well as cod liver oil. (A list of where to obtain these supplements can be found at the end of the chapter.) CCLI also recommends following the guidelines of the Weston A. Price Foundation[6] for optimal fertility nutrition.

On Hormones

In addition to taking vitamins and dietary supplements, some fertility treatments may involve taking hormones. These medications have various side effects, and many women feel like they are having an out-of-body experience when they take all these medications.

While our friend Alice and her husband were pursuing infertility treatments, Alice had injectable hormones administered that had an adverse effect on her. She remembers going into a rage, throwing things at her husband and screaming at him, which was out of the norm for her, since she is normally an even-keeled person. Her husband even wondered if the reason they were not conceiving was because of reactions like that. But they later realized that it was an adverse reaction to all the fertility drugs she was taking that caused her to feel and react this way. As a result, they decided to stop these hormone treatments. This is one example of how each person responds differently to various medications, so it is important to always be aware of possible side effects.

Mounting Costs

I wish I could honestly say that costs did not factor into all of the treatment considerations, but they did for us. We had high insurance deductibles to meet, which meant that, in addition to our insurance premium, we were paying for tests and procedures and the costs went up and up. Our budget for health care was always just for our health insurance before we began our journey with infertility, but now we constantly get bills for tests that have been run, doctors whom we've visited, and labs that have been drawn. It has taken a toll on our finances as well, and one begins to question whether this is what God wants. I know there was a point when I was just completely exhausted from all of it. I grew tired of all the treatments—the needles, the tests, the pills, and so forth. Doctors' offices, which were places I rarely visited before infertility, became places often frequented with different opinions expressed and no solutions to the enigma of what was happening.

It can also be difficult to fight with insurance companies for coverage, and once again, I learned I needed to stand up for myself. I had to learn to ask doctors to code visits for the underlying problem or potential problem—such as endometriosis or menstrual disorder—rather than infertility because infertility is not covered by insurance, though it is a disease. At one point I found myself questioning the Catholic treatment options because I felt my treatment options were limited due to our particular diagnoses, and I was worried about the costs. My insurance did not cover these treatments, and the estimates I received were tens of thousands of dollars. I questioned whether we should pursue those treatments that had no guarantees or use the same money to pursue adoption. As these questions surfaced, I took refuge in my faith, in my God.

It may be best to discuss your financial limits ahead of time if you can. Infertility is expensive to treat, and it helps to discuss with your spouse what you can realistically afford to spend. Keeping the lines of communication open while you're going through it can also help. Costs for potential treatments should also be discussed with doctors up front.

The Waiting Game

In addition to mounting costs, mounting worry also builds as the infertility journey progresses and the sense of waiting is heightened—waiting for test results, for a doctor's assessment of our situation, and for the infamous "two-week wait" (the two weeks between potential conception and being able to take a pregnancy test). But through this wait, it helps to recall Matthew 6:27: "Can any of you by worrying add a single moment to your life-span?"

Often the hardest part of anything is the wait. There were many months when the wait was full of hope, and this made the disappointment seem all the more bitter. This growing disappointment and worry begs the question, Just how much should one pursue? Also, to what extent does a Catholic have an obligation to pursue treatment?

Fertility is a finite period, and this factored into our decision. The catechism says, "The Gospel shows that physical sterility is not an absolute evil. Spouses who still suffer from infertility after exhausting legitimate medical procedures should unite themselves with the Lord's Cross, the source of all spiritual fecundity. They can give expression to their generosity by adopting abandoned children or performing demanding services for others" (*CCC* 2379).

When I read the part that says "after exhausting legitimate medical procedures," I really questioned whether I needed to proceed with what was for us the last treatment—a laparoscopy. I was on the fence about the procedure for months but finally came to the point where a decision needed to be made, and I felt this part of the catechism spoke to me that we needed to strongly consider exhausting this last possibility, if not now possibly at a later point.

We may find ourselves questioning the timing of our decisions, but scripture offers comfort and hope for these times:

There is an appointed time for everything, and a time for every affair under the heavens.

A time to be born, and a time to die;
> a time to plant, and a time to uproot the plant.

A time to kill, and a time to heal;
> a time to tear down, and a time to build.

A time to weep, and a time to laugh;
> a time to mourn, and a time to dance.

A time to scatter stones, and a time to gather them;
> a time to embrace, and a time to be far from embraces.

A time to seek, and a time to lose;
> a time to keep, and a time to cast away.

A time to rend, and a time to sew;
> a time to be silent, and a time to speak.

A time to love, and a time to hate;
> a time of war, and a time of peace.

Ecclesiastes 3:1–15

How Many Opinions to Seek

Should we explore the health concerns and at least get to the bottom of what is wrong? Is there a point at which you may have too many differing opinions? At this point, trusting the Holy Spirit and his guidance is key. The tools of discernment discussed in chapter 5 can help.

After two and a half years of infertility, we had consulted about a dozen doctors between the two of us, and it was overwhelming. Having too many opinions was hard to deal with at times. When I have been in the midst of discerning whether or not to seek additional opinions, I have always needed to remind myself of the call we all have to live in mystery. Though society makes us feel that we need definitive answers—that we have a right to the answers—that is not the case. We are tempted by the same evil spirit that tempted Adam and Eve and whispers in our ear that we are gods. Infertility and the treatments that are allowed by the Catholic Church can actually help us to become grounded in our proper place and remind us that God is in control.

For instance, in our case of secondary infertility it was abundantly clear that we believed children would be given to us whenever we wanted, especially because when we had conceived previously we had not done anything out of the ordinary. But then after years of treatments and prayers, we knew that it was only God who could change the course of events if he saw fit. We weren't going to do anything different. We were forced to abandon ourselves to God's will. This is something that we are called to do regardless of the cross we carry, and infertility helped us learn and constantly remember, whether we wanted to or not, that we are created by God and are not gods ourselves.

I have also come to see true discipleship and abandonment in friends of ours who traveled the road of infertility before us and came to the decision that they were called to be parents through adoption. In their adoption process, there were several times where they knew that their profile was being shown to potential birth mothers, and they asked for prayers. When they were not chosen, they peacefully relied on their faith in knowing God had already chosen their child for them. Their witness of abandonment to God's will challenged me to do the same.

Staying Organized and Informed

In addition to being an advocate for oneself, one also needs to be as informed and organized as possible. As our journey continued, the mound of papers seemed to grow taller and taller as more tests and charts were added. It was important to keep everything organized. I created folders for all the tests and kept all the correspondence with the doctors in a folder as well. I also kept digital copies of all the medical records, which was convenient because it allowed me to access the records from anywhere easily. It takes time to be informed and to be organized. Creating my monthly fertility cycle charts to be sent for review seemed to take me so long, and I would grow frustrated because this became like a second job to add to my already lengthy list of responsibilities. It was not something I wanted to face in the first place, and then for it to be so time-consuming made it all the more frustrating.

Based on our experience, I encourage you to ask questions and take notes when talking to your doctor. Note taking was particularly important for me because there was no other way I could remember all the medicines I had to take or how to take them. It also allowed me time to go back to see if I properly understood or needed clarification.

One of the answers to the prayers of many faithful Catholics is the advances in science that have allowed us to understand God's gift of fertility in a much deeper way. As an NFP teacher, I always tell my students that one of the best perks of NFP is learning how intricate and complex our bodies are. I took an advanced placement biology course in high school and even took biology in college, but I never learned about the workings of my body the way I have through NFP. I also firmly believe that my husband and I were not as tempted by Assisted Reproductive Technologies (ARTs) as we could have been had we not known as much about our bodies as we did. Through our study of NFP and Theology of the Body, we learned to respect God's creation in a new and profound way. We saw the bigger picture of God's design in our gender differences and appreciated the messages and signs our bodies gave us.

Unexplained Infertility

Sometimes, no matter how many medical opinions we seek out, the result can end up being an unexplained reason for infertility. Undergoing a battery of tests only to be told that nothing can be found is hard because if there are no identifiable causes or potential causes of infertility, there is nothing to treat, no plan of action. As Angelique described in chapter 1, getting a diagnosis of unexplained infertility can lead to mixed feelings:

> Though we were happy to know that our tests checked out okay, it was hard to know how to proceed. It's frustrating to see that conception isn't taking place and yet there

seemingly isn't any reason for it. Insemination or IVF
are the treatments typically recommended in these situations, but that was not an option for us. Others' implications of it potentially being psychological are particularly
hard and add fuel to the annoying "just relax" comments.
Unexplained infertility led us to God to discern whether
to continue trying while waiting on his timing or perhaps
pursue another avenue such as adoption.

The key is to continue to pray, asking God for guidance
and discerning with your spouse how to proceed. The following poem, which is often attributed to Archbishop Fulton
Sheen, offers words of wisdom in times of distrust: "Trust him
when dark doubts assail thee; trust him when trust is small.
Trust him when simply to trust him is the hardest thing of all."

Treating the Emotional Aspect of Infertility

One of the most difficult aspects of infertility is the impact
it has on your emotional health. This is often ignored by doctors who are trying to figure out what is wrong physically. The
stress and emotions may go unrecognized by the patient until
a boiling point is reached. The inability to conceive can lead
to a wide spectrum of emotions, ranging from slight stress to
overt depression and feelings of worthlessness for not being
able to achieve what the body was designed to do.

It is extremely important to seek comprehensive treatment for infertility, including psychological care. Although
daily prayer is key, other forms of support may be needed. A
good counselor can offer coping strategies that will help you
in difficult situations, such as events where there will be many
children or pregnant women in attendance. A support group
may also offer spiritual healing. If you begin to note symptoms such as lack of interest in activities that you previously
enjoyed, inability to sleep, feelings of guilt, lack of energy, or
decreased appetite, bring them to the attention of your doctor
or seek counseling, as they may be signs of depression.

Seeking comprehensive Catholic medical care for our
infertility means going against the grain of what mainstream

society is offering us and, though liberating, can be challenging as well. Invoking Our Lady of Good Counsel can help strengthen our resolve to uphold human dignity while also hopefully finding healing for the underlying causes of our infertility through Catholic treatment.

Prayer for the Intercession of Our Lady of Good Counsel

Holy Virgin, moved by the painful uncertainty we experience in seeking and acquiring the true and the good, we invoke you as Mother of Good Counsel. Please come to our aid and obtain for us from your Divine Son the love of virtue and the strength to choose, in these doubtful and difficult situations, the course agreeable to our salvation. Supported by your hand we shall journey without harm along the paths taught us by the word and example of Jesus our Savior. Amen.[7]

Different NFP Methods

Sympto-Thermal Method—through the observations of cervical mucus, basal body temperature, and the cervix, couples learn to identify fertile and infertile phases of their cycle. Classes are taught by couples throughout the country or you can learn at home. Contact the Couple to Couple League International:

>Couple to Couple League International, Inc. (Sympto-Thermal Method)
>(513) 471-2000 or (800) 745-8252
>www.ccli.org

Billings Ovulation Method—uses cervical mucus observations to determine a woman's fertility.

>Billings Ovulation Method Association (BOMA-USA)
>(651) 699-8139
>info@boma-usa.org
>www.boma-usa.org

The Creighton Model Fertility*Care*™ System (CrMS) is a standardized modification of the Billings Ovulation Method that analyzes cervical mucus.[8]

The Creighton Model System (NaProTECHNOLOGY)
Pope Paul VI Institute for the Study of Human Reproduction
(402) 390-6600
popepaul@popepaulvi.com
www.naprotechnology.com; www.popepaulvi.com

Marquette Model (MM)—uses a fertility monitor (a device used at home that measures hormone levels in urine to estimate the beginning and end of the time of fertility) in conjunction with observations of cervical mucus, basal body temperature, or other biological indicators of fertility.[9]

The Marquette Model (MM)
The Institute for Natural Family Planning
(414) 288-3838
nfp.marquette.edu

If you would like to learn any of these methods you should contact the individual organization responsible for promoting the method, and they will point you in the right direction.

Technologies Compatible with Catholic Teachings

1. Observation of the naturally occurring sign(s) of fertility (Natural Family Planning).[10] Timing intercourse on the days of presumed (potential) fertility for at least six months before proceeding to medical interventions.

    This is generally the first course of action and one that is prescribed by doctors regularly because it helps couples know when they are fertile and maximize the chance of achieving pregnancy. Charting may also be indicative of other medical problems that affect fertility.

2. General medical evaluation of both spouses for infertility. This includes physical exams and blood tests to check for hormone levels.

3. Postcoital test to assess sperm number and viability in "fertile-type" mucus. These tests are undertaken after normal intercourse. These tests are done to see if the mucus is potentially hostile to the sperm and not providing the sperm the necessary nutrients to allow for conception. The cervical mucus is examined for various features such as stretchiness, ferning, and so forth, and they check for the sperm within the mucus.

   Please keep in mind this test has been eliminated from most standard workups.

4. Appropriate evaluation and treatment of male factor deficiency. Seminal fluid samples can be obtained from a nonlubricated, perforated condom after normal intercourse. You must speak to the lab to indicate that this is the way you would like to perform this test in lieu of masturbation to obtain a sperm sample. A perforated condom allows for sperm to potentially enter the vagina and is therefore not being used as a contraceptive but rather as a device to collect the sample for analysis while allowing for new life to be formed potentially. Treatment may include surgery to repair a varicocele, for example. This is to restore the male's health.

5. Assessment of uterine and tubal structural competence by imaging techniques (e.g., ultrasound, hysterosalpingogram, etc.). These tests allow doctors to see if there are blockages in the fallopian tubes, for example, and some of the tests are therapeutic as well. A hysterosalpingogram can remove any small blockage through the procedure itself; the liquid/dye used to see the organs can remove any blockage.

6. Appropriate medical treatment of ovulatory dysfunction. For example, Clomid or clomi atment that helps ovulation and the quality of the follicles produced.

   Many of the drugs used to overcome infertility help the woman's body do what it is naturally supposed to do. Progesterone

Advantages of Catholic Treatment

- Medically safe
- Morally acceptable
- Promotes shared responsibility and strengthens marriage
- Provides knowledge of a woman's body
- Tries to address the causes of infertility
- Allows greater collaboration between physician and patient

supplements are another common prescription for infertility. These supplements are given to prevent potential miscarriage. Through the use of medications, doctors can also help treat polycystic ovary syndrome (PCOS), a common cause of infertility.

7. Appropriate (usually surgical) correction of mechanical blocks to tubal patency (the state of being open). This is an acceptable treatment because it tries to restore the body to the way it should be. This can be laparoscopy or hysteroscopies, for example.

Further Reading

Chavarro, Jorge. *The Fertility Diet*. New York: McGraw-Hill, 2008.
A book providing nutritional recommendations for maximizing fertility.

Falcone, Tommaso, and Tanya R. Falcone. *The Cleveland Clinic Guide to Infertility*. New York: Kaplan, 2009.
An easy-to-understand explanation of many of the issues you will face with infertility.

Pope Paul VI Institute. "Infertility: A Couple's Struggle." Accessed September 16, 2011. www.catholicinfertility.org.
Support and treatment options for Catholics dealing with infertility.

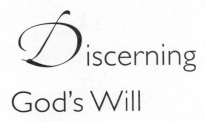
Discerning
God's Will

To love God is to will what He wills.

Blessed Charles de Foucauld

For so long during my infertility journey, I just wanted to do what God wanted—to do his will—but I couldn't figure out what that was. I used to think that God's will was like a blueprint or a master plan that I needed to figure out. It was as if I needed to guess at what he wanted for my life, and I was afraid of choosing the wrong path. I would obsess over doing God's will as if God had a concrete choice for me in every decision I made, and all I could do was hope I was choosing what God wanted me to choose.

The problem with this idea is that it precludes the possibility of free will. If we truly believe in free will, then we cannot also believe that God has his own concrete will for us. God's will is not something God wants *for* us but rather something God wants *from* us. God's will is simply that which leads us closer to him. It's not a magic formula we need to figure out.

We are free to choose his love and in that way choose the best thing for ourselves and for our families. God allows us to make decisions to see how we can best accomplish this. Fortunately, there are tools we can use to help us choose to follow God's will, to choose that which leads us closer to him. In our faith tradition, we call this discernment.

Choose Wisely

We spend our lives making decisions, some mundane—like what we're going to wear today or what flavor of coffee we will have. Others are a little more life altering, like our vocations. In our walk as Christians, we are faced with a number of options, all of which are attractive, and we are called to sift through these options to discover what might be the "best Christian response."[1] What should I do? Which option is best? How do I even go about deciding this? These decisions and choices are what help define our walk with Christ.

The word *discernment* is often considered synonymous with decision making, and though discernment does facilitate our decision making, it is so much more than simply making choices. In the discernment process, we are drawn closer to God by choosing to do his will. In this chapter, you will learn helpful tools for discernment as you confront the many (and often overwhelming) decisions that arise with infertility, including if and how to test, whether to pursue fertility treatments (and how far to go), and whether to pursue adoption. Though this chapter aims at helping us to make decisions related to infertility, the tools of discernment outlined can be used to choose God in all areas of our lives.

Many Catholic authors have written on the subject of discernment, but St. Ignatius of Loyola is perhaps the most well-known writer to elaborate upon the concept in his Spiritual Exercises (SE), where he suggests that the best way for us to make a life-changing decision is through the "discernment of spirits" (SE 178–83). Discernment is a choice between two courses of action, both of which are morally good. It might be much easier if our choice was simply between a good and an evil, since as Christians, we know that evil is never really an option and thus it is readily discarded.

We have learned from the time we were young that we should never knowingly choose wrong. So in the case of infertility, a proper discernment cannot be made, for example, between Catholic treatments, which are licit, and in vitro fertilization, which is illicit. The Christian may only choose between two (or more) good, moral options. We are called to the *magis*, a Latin term that St. Ignatius often used that loosely means "the greater good."

Discernment is not just picking one thing over another; it is a process of analyzing our choices one by one and finding how they align with our goals. If deciding between two different job opportunities, for example, one would have to pick one over the other. But in the case of infertility, it is possible that when discerning each choice individually, God may be calling a couple to pursue two options simultaneously, for example, pursuing treatment *and* adoption. We must be open to whatever outcome we are being called, provided the outcome(s) are in conformity with Church teaching. "Discernment is at the heart of discipleship because when we walk a disciple's path, we are constantly faced with changing situations in which we have to discover how to be faithful to the Gospel and the leading of the Spirit, and true to ourselves."[2] This is certainly true for infertility, as it is a "changing situation"—or more appropriately, a situation that changes us—in which we are still called to be faithful to the Gospel.

The purpose of discernment is not as much about making decisions as it is about directing our thoughts and feelings toward loving God with all your heart, all your being, all your strength, and with all your mind, and toward loving your neighbor as yourself (Lk 10:27). Discernment may involve asking for directions. Even Jesus' closest companions had to ask him for directions. Good old doubting Thomas asked Jesus, "Master, we do not know where you are going; how can we know the way?" (Jn 14:5).

Some of the choices we make are final (such as marriage or a religious vocation), and others have a more limited time frame, but all of our important decisions should direct us toward God. To Ignatius, who sets forth the goal of our lives in the Principle and Foundation (found in chapter 2), we are created by God to praise, reverence, and serve God. Thus it follows that, in any decision, we must consider the praise, reverence, and service of God above all so that our decisions help us attain this goal for our lives. And that's why it's so important to make good decisions.

In the end, discernment can be simplified by asking the question, "What is the more loving or life-giving thing to do?"

Freedom and Indifference

In the Principle and Foundation, Ignatius says, "As long as we are allowed free choice, we must make ourselves indifferent to all created things" (SE 23). Indifference does not equal apathy. According to St. Ignatius, indifference means standing "as a balance at equilibrium, without leaning to one side or the other" (SE 15). If I am trying to decide between continuing to pursue Catholic treatment options or stopping treatment altogether, I cannot enter the formal discernment process hoping and praying that the outcome is to continue treatment, for instance, because then I may bias the discernment. Similarly, the Principle and Foundation says we should not "prefer health to sickness"—or, in this case, fertility to infertility. As difficult as it is, we should make ourselves indifferent to whether or not we have a child. We should pray for God to grant us the grace of indifference so that we may be open to the outcome toward which God is guiding us.

By calling for indifference, Ignatius calls us to desire to be influenced by God's guidance throughout the discernment process. Passionate indifference requires that we be so passionate about loving God that we do not have a preference for the means that best lead us there. This is incredibly difficult since essentially it means that we cannot have any attachments—material or emotional. However, the more freedom we have from attachments, the more open we become to finding where he is truly calling us and the more freedom we have to love passionately, as Jesus did.

Freedom can feel like a burden once we realize there are no blueprints or instructions in God's mind that we must blindly follow. God may seem harshly mute when we ask him to reveal his will for us. But God wants to share with us his divine compassion by calling us to choose whatever we want, provided we are motivated by our love for him.

As our loving creator, God knows the depths of our hearts better than we do. Only he can know what will bring us the most joy and what will make us feel most complete. It is therefore in our best interest to ask God for his help when we make a decision—not because we are trying to guess what he wants for us but because he knows what our hearts truly desire. Remember that God loves us and wants us to share in his joy and love.

Before even approaching a decision, we must first have inner freedom, which is rooted in the freely given love of God. When we love God in return, we set out to share the good, the truth, the unity, and the beauty that the Lord, our Creator, has put in us freely.

When I was in elementary school, I used to love to read Choose Your Own Adventure books, which are a series of books where each page offers the reader an opportunity to choose where she's going next. Will I choose to take the mine car out of the abandoned mine? If so, I will turn to page 40 to continue my adventure. If I choose to try to climb out using a rope, I turn to page 48 and keep reading from there. This analogy is the best way for me to understand freedom in terms of making a decision in Christ. We can look at our lives as having a Master Author who single-handedly determines the outcome and ending of our books. Or we can view our lives as a Choose Your Own Adventure book, where there is indeed an Author but one who gives us choices and trusts in our ability and will to freely choose life with him as our ultimate adventure.

We should pray for an increased awareness of the things that are blocking us from this kind of freedom, and we must honestly admit our attachments or dependencies. Do not underestimate the role sin plays in the discernment process. Nothing keeps us from true inner freedom more than sin. The more we sin and make excuses for our sins, the more our vision of God becomes obstructed. It is a good idea to have a sincere confession prior to discerning. In the process of attaining inner freedom prior to making a decision, we should also consider questions like, How influential are my emotions like fear or love? Do I concern myself too much with what others will think or with the desire to be successful? If so, bringing these to prayer and offering up our attachments or fears will help make a good discernment.

Four prerequisites for a good discernment:

1. ready to move in any direction God wants, therefore radically free (indifference);

2. open to sharing all that God has given him or her, therefore radically generous;

3. willing to suffer if God's will requires it, therefore radically patient; and

4. questing for union with God in prayer, therefore radically spiritual.[3]

Steps of Ignatian Discernment

Spiritual Exercises 178–83

In his Spiritual Exercises, St. Ignatius explains in detail how to discern. It can be a little complex at times, with a vast number of rules, but below is a synthesized version of his rules of discernment that have aided us in making important decisions in our lives.

For each step, I will give concrete examples from the discernment my husband and I made while we were facing infertility. We still have the notebooks we used to do this discernment, and it has served us well to look back on it and see how God worked through that process to guide us to adopt our son. I share our own personal discernment in order to show how the discernment process works. God calls each of us in different ways and through different means. Your own discernment process and outcome need not resemble ours.

1. *Identify the decision that needs to be made and formulate a question.*
   Even though Ignatian spirituality is my personal charism and
   I had discerned things in the past, I decided to read up on discernment before we started, especially since my husband and I
   were discerning how to proceed together.[4] I read one book that
   suggested that, when discerning a number of things, we should
   take each question individually so as not to confuse the process.

   After experiencing about one year of infertility, we had read
   up on both NaProTECHNOLOGY and adoption, and for whatever reason, we felt God was prompting us to adopt, but we
   weren't completely sure yet. So the first question we brought
   forth to our discernment was "Are we called to adopt?"

   We decided on a date when we were both free (a Saturday afternoon—the discernment ended up running into Sunday morning as well!) and began our discernment with that
   question.

2. *Be indifferent to the end result. Remember that the goal is to praise,
   reverence, and serve God.*
   My husband and I talked about the fears and attachments we
   each had before starting to discern. Things like desiring to bear
   a child biologically and fear of the unknown were brought to
   light. Talking them through in the weeks before we discerned
   helped us to be able to offer them up in order to be indifferent
   to the outcome.

3. *Pray for God's guidance during the discernment.*
   We sat on our living room couch that Saturday afternoon, and
   my husband led us by praying for God to guide our discernment. He offered up any personal reservations and fears and
   asked for God's will to be done. I then also prayed out loud for
   my own attachments and for God to help us to choose the most
   life-giving option. Starting out with a prayer and asking for God's
   grace welcomed the Holy Spirit into the process.

4. *Using your head and your heart, create a list of pros and cons of
   the different outcomes.*
   When doing a communal discernment where more than one
   person is involved, you may opt to do individual pro-con lists
   and then come together to discuss it and create one joint list; or

you may prefer to do just one pro-con list. Either is acceptable. My husband and I opted to do it individually first to not bias the other. We both sat on the same couch and individually answered the question "Are we called to adopt?" by formulating our own pro-con lists with our thoughts and feelings on the subject, and when we were each done, we shared our lists and created one consolidated pro-con list.

I remember reading beforehand that no pro or con was too silly or insignificant to be taken into consideration, so even the most mundane things found their way to the list. Our lists were very detailed. That way, we knew we were both being completely honest with ourselves and with one another.

5. *Reflect on pros and cons, becoming aware of where you feel consolation and desolation (discussed in the next section). Make a decision.*
    When we came together to share our pro-con lists, it was obvious that the pros of adopting outweighed the cons. Even so, it's important to remember that it's not so much the number of pros versus cons that should be considered; each individual pro and con should be looked at in terms of its value or importance to the decision.

    For any con or area of concern or questions, we tried to formulate an answer or solution together to ensure there was no area that was insurmountable. For example, the cost of adoption was a major con for both of us, but when we discussed it, possible solutions we came up with were the adoption tax credit (discussed further in chapter 12) and the fact that my husband's employer at the time offered adoption assistance grants for employees.

    Based on the consolation we both felt, we decided we were being called to adopt.

6. *Be thankful to God for accompanying you in this discernment, and pray without delay to confirm your decision.*
    Immediately after finishing your discernment process, take a moment to thank God for the grace to discern with him. St. Ignatius also encourages discerners to pray before Jesus to confirm their decisions, be it before the Blessed Sacrament or at Mass.

Since we concluded our adoption discernment on a Sunday, we went to our regular evening Mass and brought our decision before the Lord on the altar. I must confess that, when we saw the priest who was celebrating the Mass that evening, we were a little disappointed because, though he is a kind man and a good priest, he was not known to be the best homilist. Nevertheless, we knelt before the Mass began to ask God to please confirm our decision to adopt a child. During that Mass, we learned never to underestimate the power of God to speak in unexpected ways!

The Gospel that evening happened to be Matthew 14:22–33, when Peter walks on water. "Take courage, it is I," Jesus tells his friends. "Do not be afraid." Peter began walking on the water toward Jesus, but when he felt how strong the wind was he began to doubt he could do it and started to sink, crying out to Jesus to save him. I imagine Jesus' teasing smile as he grabs hold of Peter's hand and tells him, "O you of little faith, why did you doubt?"

I can't say I remember anything specific from that homily— I remember squeezing my husband's hand really tight while the Gospel was being read—but I do remember feeling blown away (like St. Peter, maybe?) by how it spoke to the core of trusting in Jesus in our call to adopt a child. When we married, the thought of adopting a child was about as likely as us walking on water, but God makes the impossible possible. Needless to say, the decision to adopt that we had made just hours earlier was confirmed at that Mass.

After discerning the initial question of whether we were being called to adopt, we discerned other questions, such as "Are we being called to adopt domestically or internationally?" (the answer was internationally); "From which country?" (we had three different options and felt called to adopt from Vietnam); and "Which agency should we use?" (after researching many options and spending hours on the phone interviewing agencies, we narrowed it down to three; we brought these three into the discernment process and narrowed it down using our pro-con lists).

Our friend Nora created a great user-friendly cheat sheet for discernment that comes directly from the Spiritual Exercises. You can find that at the end of this chapter.

Consolation and Desolation

In a world of noise and constant distraction, it is hard to hear God's voice sometimes. I often have to remind myself of how it was that Elijah came to hear God's voice. It was not in the strong and heavy wind, it was not in the earthquake, it was not in the fire: it was in a tiny whisper (1 Kgs 19:11–13). I tend to look for the fireworks sometimes instead of quieting myself to hear the more subtle ways that God speaks to me.

What is the voice of God? It is that which brings peace, comfort, and stillness to your soul. Ignatius calls this consolation (SE 316). Consolation brings us closer to God, helps us to be less centered upon ourselves, and draws us to open out to others in generosity, service, and love. Consolation is what we experience when our deepest desire to serve God is aligned with our decision.

Desolation is the opposite of consolation (SE 317). The voice of the evil spirit, in contrast, is that which brings anxiety, pain, and restlessness to your soul. Ignatius called this desolation. Desolation draws us away from God and leads us to be self-centered, closed, and unconcerned about God or other people.[5]

We need to test the spirits, test those feelings that are vying for our attention in order to see whether we feel consolation or desolation in the face of a decision. We may not hear an actual voice with a distinct verbal message, but we will be moved to experience either consolation or desolation. These stirrings are what will ultimately confirm our decision or will lead us to reexamine our choice.

It is important to realize that consolation and desolation do not equate to happy and sad feelings, respectively. A poor decision can still lead to transient feelings of happiness, much like a good decision can lead to doubt, fear, and stifling feelings. What's important is to realize which of these stirrings of the soul persist after the decision has been made. It's not about how we feel in the moment but more about which feeling lasts beyond the initial gladness of having made a decision, whether good or bad.

In our own adoption decision, we received a tremendous amount of consolation about the decision to adopt, so we jumped in and immediately started the process to adopt. But then a month into the process, we found out we were pregnant, and we (shamefully and selfishly) started to doubt and question our decision to adopt, despite how strongly we had felt consolation. Our own fears started to take over as we wondered how we'd handle two young babies at once; consequently, we thought maybe the best option was to simply postpone the adoption until a future point.

When we have doubts, Ignatius encourages us to discuss the matter with a trusted spiritual companion. Because we are all liable to self-deception, we need help to be objective and honest. God often speaks to us through the wisdom of others. In mentioning our fears and thoughts of postponing the adoption with a few people, including some close friends and the priest who married us, it was a very strong wakeup call that, in discerning to adopt and feeling that calling so strongly from God, we already had a child out there and we couldn't give up on this child just because I happened to become pregnant. It was in fact a blessing (wasn't it what we had wanted for so long?) and not something to be feared or avoided.

Sometimes evil is very deceptive because we might have easily confused these doubts with desolation, but through the help of these spiritual companions, we realized that the thought of postponing didn't give us consolation and so we proceeded with the process. These companions who challenged us were truly the voice of God for us because, if we had listened to the fear, we wouldn't have our oldest son, Emmanuel, who is a blessing beyond words. We couldn't imagine our lives without him.

The thing to keep in mind is that desolation never comes from God. If a particular option in your decision making brings you desolation—not sadness, fear, or doubt, which are normal, but actual desolation—it cannot be from God. You can safely discard this option and proceed. Evil wants one of two things. Either it wants you to quit doing the good that you are doing (which would have been the case if we had postponed the adoption), or it wants you to be desolate even though you are living a good life. If desolation is what you feel, you must keep the process open until you can arrive at a decision that head and heart can jointly embrace.

The tricky part about discernment is consolation, because consolation can either come from God or from the evil spirit. The voice of God may lead you to feel consolation to help you confirm and feel love and truth in your decision. However, since the evil spirit is a great deceiver, this spirit may also lead you to feel consolation in a decision initially. You may genuinely choose something because you think it is what will bring the most joy, hope, and peace. But this may be a trap for the evil spirit to enter your soul and later turn your seemingly wonderful decision into a path that will separate you from God.

Unfortunately, I think this is sometimes the case when Catholic couples know full well what the Church's teachings are and still choose in vitro fertilization (IVF). They may not have entered into a formal discernment process to arrive at the decision, but they may justify the decision to pursue IVF saying they feel peace and happiness in their decision. Yes, having a child is good and a blessing, but the way we go about that can be immoral and could be a path that leads away from God.

So how can you know whether your consolation is coming from God or from the evil spirit? It takes much prayer and practice to learn how to be a good discerner. It is important to receive confirmation of each decision, Ignatius says, by attending Mass or praying before the Blessed Sacrament. Additionally, it is important to realize which stirrings persist in your soul, as mentioned previously. The consolation you receive from God will always console. Even when sad feelings come about from your decision, consolation will persist

through the difficult feelings. In contrast, consolation from
the evil spirit will eventually turn into desolation. It's kind of
like athletes who must learn to distinguish between the good
pain that comes from stretching beyond the norm and bad
pain that comes from injury or overexertion.

We should never change our decision in times of desolation. We must be patient and wait until what may appear to
be desolation subsides. If it persists, pray for enlightenment;
God will guide you to reevaluate your decision if consolation
does not return to you.

Three States of the Soul

Ignatius describes three ways in which God can guide
people faced with choice. These are what he calls the three
states of the soul during decision making (SE 175–177):

1. *God overwhelms us with certainty about our decision. This is done
   in a way that precludes all doubt.* (SE 175) Ignatius uses the example of St. Paul and St. Matthew to illustrate this kind of guidance.
   In this situation, everything points in one direction, there is no
   doubt, and it makes the choice unambiguously clear.

Rarely will we experience consolation that precludes all
doubt. Our hearts will be illuminated and filled with God's
love so we cannot question the presence of our Creator in
our discernment. This is an amazing gift, but it hardly ever
happens! For most of us, God doesn't cause us to fall off a
horse and become temporarily blind so that we hear his voice
calling us. God gives us the ability to think and feel—both
of these come from him, and both of these are tools we can
use to illuminate our decisions. So the next state of the soul
involves emotions as indicators of God's guidance.

2. *We rely on our affectivity and emotions—consolation and desolation—to detect God's influence regarding the decision to be made.*
   (SE 176) This is what makes our decisions very personal. Have
   you ever made a decision that defied all logic and everyone
   questioned—even you—only to find that it was the best decision
   you ever made? If you have, it's probably because your heart

had the final word in that decision. Many of us approach choices only with our brains, and we put our hearts aside because we are trying to make the most logical choice. We fear that our hearts may steer us wrong. But God wants us to include our feelings to make a decision, too.

The term "heart" is a traditional image for a way of perceiving, feeling, and loving that engages the total person. When making a decision about infertility, we have to listen to our hearts. We have to allow God to put a divine stethoscope to our hearts to hear our inner longings to be parents. A heart-centered approach to discernment is holistic. Like the hokey pokey dance, which invites us to "put your whole self in," holistic discernment invites us to put our whole self into the process. We have to harmonize the head and the heart and use both to make decisions. Going with our heart doesn't mean we can put our intellect aside completely, either. But it means if we are so logical that we ignore our heart's desires, we will experience great pain from our decisions.

3. *We rely on our intellect and reasoning while our soul is at peace in order to detect God's guiding influence.* (SE 177) Our mind is the first tool we use when we make decisions. Most of us think quite a bit about the pros and the cons of each option we are questioning. God gives us our minds so we may use them as our initial filters to "screen" our options. This is what gives us our ability to know right from wrong and to weigh our values against our options.

For me, the most important role our intellect plays in the process of discernment is that of enlightening me to the most life-giving option. It helps to ask the question "Is this choice the more loving thing to do at this moment in my life?" It's about choosing that which you feel will bring blessings, love, and the sense of God's life heightened in you. When you work with your intellect, you list the facts and analyze how the particular option fits in with the pattern of God's action in your life.

Challenges to Discernment

Discernment works. It is a great method for being able to get some clarity on the challenging decisions we need to make while journeying through infertility. That said, it's understandable to fear it as well. It's natural to be afraid of what God is going to ask of us when we truly try to listen to his voice. A friend of mine used to always say that holiness lies outside of our comfort zones, and sometimes stepping out of what we know is precisely what God asks of us. Unfortunately, though, fears and doubts can paralyze us and cause us to procrastinate in making important decisions.

Sometimes when we are making decisions, we are afraid to invite God into the decision-making process because we are afraid he is going to want something for us that we don't want for ourselves. We shouldn't think that way. God is such a loving Father, and we cannot even imagine the kind of joy that he wants for us. Don't be afraid to tell God what you want—your own will (even though he already knows). This will help you not to feel like it's your will against his and will help you find peace. He loves us beyond measure and wants to guide us with the gifts of consolation and desolation. Even though it is tough work to make the time to sift through our fears and feelings in discernment, the end result is worth it.

As Christians, we are called to live boldly and decisively. We must act, even though our carefully discerned decisions may be tinged with some uncertainty. We are called to live out our decision with courage, hope, and trust. This requires us to trust in God and to decide, even in the absence of certitude.

A well-discerned choice can entail enduring periods of struggle and pain while at the same time be supported by a deep sense of God's presence and love. We are called to trust in God's power at work bringing good out of everything. As St. Paul says in Romans, "We know that all things work together for good for those who love God, who are called according to his purpose" (8:28).

In the same way that it is normal to experience some fear prior to discerning, it is normal to experience it after discerning as well. Doubts can creep up after making a decision and beginning to act on it. As I said, our doubts arose after becoming pregnant one month into the adoption process, but in listening to the voice of God encouraging us with the lasting consolation we felt amidst the doubts, we know we made the right decision without a shadow of a doubt. The important thing is to focus on the sentiment that lasts.

And what if you and your spouse discern how to proceed along the infertility journey and you find you're not on the same page? What if one wants to continue to pursue treatments and the other doesn't? One cannot force another to do something against his or her will any more than God forces us to do his will. Everyone has free will, and just because one person is not ready to act or move does not mean they won't be ready later on. After all, it is God's time that is best. Or perhaps God is speaking through one spouse in trying to guide the other. Either way, frustration may result at not being on the same page, but we must remember that very few decisions are final. There is always an opportunity to rediscern in the future.

Occasionally, we will make the wrong choice. Whenever this is the case, we must first pray about it. Taking an example from my own life unrelated to infertility, my husband and I once discerned to put an offer to buy a house that I was not that enthused about. Because we had been house hunting for about a year and a half and my husband liked the house, we did a discernment together on whether or not to put an offer on the house. Though the outcome of the discernment indicated that we should make an offer (based on the intellectual pro-con portion of the discernment and our initial consolation), we decided to wait a little while to see how we felt about the decision—what our hearts said about it. In the end, we never really felt consolation; more like resignation! We never felt comfortable putting an offer on that house and

instead decided to wait. We ended up finding a house down
the line that was a better fit for our family.

In all circumstances, no matter what we decide, it is well
to remember that there is nothing in this world that will
change God's desire to bless us with his grace. We just need
to first trust in that grace, and this is what discernment is
really about. It's not about formulas and pros versus cons—it's
about trusting that God knows our desire to make a choice
that is good, loving, and life giving, and that he will help us
figure out the way. God lovingly made us in his image, and he
equipped us with everything we need to hear his voice, but
we must open our hearts to him. If we pray with open hearts,
we will learn to listen to the voice of God.

> More than ever I find myself in the hands of God. This is
> what I have wanted all my life from my youth. But now
> there is a difference; the initiative is entirely with God. It
> is indeed a profound spiritual experience to know and
> feel myself so totally in God's hands.
>
> *Pedro Arrupe*

Discernment Worksheet

1. Use your intellect to do this portion:

Pros	Cons

2. Use your affectivity (feelings) to do this portion (analyze the column that best fits your decision):

When I think about this option, the predominant feelings that come to mind are

Consolation	Desolation
Increase in Faith	Lack of Faith
Hope	Hopelessness
Joy	Sadness
Closeness to God	Separation from God
Peace	Restlessness

Repeat steps 1 and 2 for each option in question. Remember that discernment is not just deciding two options but rather a process of analyzing each different option separately.

3. After making your decision, reflect upon your feelings, and see if they fall under the consolation or desolation categories. Do *not* change your decision if you begin to doubt and have some feelings of desolation. It is normal to experience difficult feelings following an important decision. Wait to see if these feelings subside with time. If they do not, then you will have to reevaluate your discernment.

If you are still undecided after doing these first three steps, use any of these methods (alone or in combination):

*   Measure your option in terms of the Principle and Foundation.

*   Pray.

*   Imagine a friend coming to us for help in making a choice similar to the one we are facing. We should listen carefully to what we counsel this person to do and then follow our own advice.

*   Think about your option as if you were on your deathbed—what path would you have wanted to take?

*   Imagine living with a choice for a set period of time, and see which choice gives more peace.

*   Reflect about your option as if you were at the gates of heaven— would you change it?

*   Think about which option is the most loving.

$\mathcal{T}$he Cross
of Infertility

Love and follow Christ! If the path becomes difficult at
times and you are overcome by fatigue, rest in the shade
of prayer.

Blessed John Paul II

Few transitions seem more difficult to a woman struggling
with infertility than that of going from desiring to bear a
child to learning to bear a cross instead. Although the journey of infertility is different for each individual, carrying this
cross is part of what God has called some of us to do as faithful
Christians. With the help of prayer and perseverance, we can
grow stronger from our efforts.

Scripture offers us wisdom that can help us grow closer to
Christ through this process. Jesus said to his disciples, "Whoever wishes to come after me must deny himself, take up his
cross, and follow me" (Mt 16:24). Here, Christ makes it clear
that three distinct steps are required: self-denial, bearing the
cross, and following/trusting him.

Self-Denial

Combating Comparisons

St. Teresa of Avila said comparison is the death of the spiritual life. How often did I compare myself to others—to the other people around me who got pregnant seemingly so easily or without "wanting" to?

At a particularly weak point in my journey, I found out that three friends were pregnant simultaneously, and it seemed like almost more than I could bear. These were women who had either tried for one month to get pregnant or weren't even trying, and here I was, after years of trying, with still no baby. Many infertile couples begin avoiding social situations (baby showers, baptisms, etc.) in order to avoid seeing babies or pregnant people. It is undoubtedly difficult to be surrounded by constant reminders of what we do not have, yet we are also called to be grateful to God for those who do.

Many times it was hard for me to ask some friends about their pregnancies and how they were feeling. In these cases, I had to make an even greater effort to ask because I had to overcome my sinful tendency with the corresponding virtue. Pride rears its ugly head on too many occasions, from feeling that a friend's good news of being pregnant needed to be told to me in a special way, to thinking we could traverse this road of infertility without God's grace to sustain us. At the blog *Lear, Kent, Fool*, Suzanne wrote,

> I would sometimes hear other Catholic moms quietly share their fears and dismay about becoming pregnant "again," "so soon." This kind of talk was difficult for me to hear, to say the least. Some days it made me want to scream. I never actually did. I just listened in silence and cried later. Many of us who have struggled with infertility have felt this way.[1]

We should also not compare our infertility journeys. One person's struggle is not worse or more legitimate because they've gone through it longer or because they've had more medical procedures, for example. Each one of us has our own journey, and we need to focus on learning and being strengthened by it. God knows how to perfect us and is using what each person needs to achieve that.

I have found that comparisons sometimes lead to a feeling of a sense of entitlement. For example, my husband and I have always done our best to follow God's laws and even began learning Natural Family Planning (NFP) before we got married, and yet so-and-so uses birth control and got pregnant right away. These comparisons did not lead to anything helpful. I learned that, when I begin to feel less than charitable, I need to try harder to be loving. Blessed John Paul II explained the gifts of the spirit in a way I can relate to. He said that a fruit takes time to mature, and at first it is not ripe and does not taste sweet. The same goes for the spiritual gifts, and these gifts will produce fruits.

When I am facing difficulties, I often recall this story of St. Teresa of Avila: Teresa was riding a donkey cart when one of the wheels fell into a ditch, launching her into the mud. She looked to heaven and exclaimed, "If this is the way you treat your friends, it is no wonder you have so few of them!" I often feel this way because I believe that Jesus is my friend, but I cannot lose sight of the fact that he is God. I have to make an effort to change my view so that I may try to glean what God wants me to learn from a situation instead of questioning why I'm in it.

Embracing Our Brokenness

A popular Indian tale called *The Broken Pot* tells the story of two pots. Each hung on one end of a pole that a water bearer carried on his neck on his way to retrieve water for his master. One pot had a crack in it, and on the trip back from retrieving the water, half of the contents would inevitably leak out of it while the other pot was intact. The pot with the crack was sad about his flaw and told the water bearer. The bearer said to the pot,

> Did you notice that there were flowers only on your side of the path, but not on the other pot's side? That's because I have always known about your flaw, and I took advantage of it. I planted flower seeds on your side of the path, and every day while we walk back from the stream, you've watered them. For two years I have been able to pick these beautiful flowers to decorate my master's table. Without you being just the way you are, he would not have this beauty to grace his house.

We can view infertility as a flaw, like the crack in the pot, but if we only focus on the crack and do not see what beauty or flowers can be born of this difficulty, we are doing the world a disservice. God will use our cracks; we simply need to trust him.

Society wants us to cover up our flaws to hide our weakness and brokenness from each other. However, denying our brokenness may discourage us from turning to God in the way we most need since he is the only one who can heal our hurt. Infertility is a brokenness that many people find very difficult to deal with. There is so much sadness out there on this topic and some of that is chronicled on the myriad of Catholic infertility blogs (some of these blogs are listed in chapter 7). One of the reasons infertility is such a struggle is because you want something that is only natural. It is natural, even instinctual, to want children. There is nothing wrong with it, and yet it is something to which God ultimately has said no at some point in our lives. It may be no, not right now, or no, forever, but for whatever reason infertility is our cross. It is also a challenge because it is a public cross to bear. Not having children is something that is out there for the world to see. This can many times lead to painful probing by people who surround us.

I was reading a devotional recently that talked about suffering. It discussed the temptation we fall into of asking "why me?" and the devotional invited us to ask ourselves "why not me?" The question struck me because I had never thought of it that way. Why not me? Why can't I carry the cross of infertility? Why can't I be the one who is an example to others? The question haunted me for quite some time, and I thought of it often in prayer. What good reason did I have for not walking the road of infertility? I know that through difficulty comes growth, but it's so comfortable not to experience difficulties and not to learn to trust completely. When we feel betrayed by God we should pray to change our cry from "why me" to "why not me." Our suffering makes us more human, better able to relate and minister to others. There is a level of compassion that can only be achieved when the suffering is shared.

In Matthew 16:15, Jesus asks, "Who do you say that I am?" We answer this question in how we live our lives. It's a question we are constantly asked and constantly answering. Others notice our actions and will see Christ in the way we respond to our suffering. How we carry our cross is an answer to Jesus' question.

The Pain of the Cross

It is interesting to think about how our concept of suffering has changed through time. In our society of instant gratification and "happy pills," suffering has become something that we reject to a great extent. People do not want to feel pain. Even our grandparents' "valley of tears" faith is lost on our generation. The early Christians knew they must suffer to enter the kingdom of God (Acts 14:22), yet we reject our suffering.

In his Second Letter to the Corinthians, Paul says, "For this slight momentary affliction is preparing for us an eternal weight of glory beyond all comparison, because we look not to the things that are seen but to things that are unseen" (2 Cor 4:17–18). We are not home yet and will not be until we are (God willing) in heaven with our Lord. Infertility is a journey, part of the travails toward our home in heaven. St. Paul reminds us that this time is only a drop in the bucket, so to speak, and is minimal compared to eternity. It is up to us to choose to view and use infertility as a tool to prepare us for our ultimate home. Maintaining a faith perspective throughout our suffering, particularly with the suffering from infertility, helps us apply purpose to our suffering.

Blessed John Paul II said, "Those who share in the suffering of Christ become worthy of this Kingdom. Through their sufferings, in a certain sense they repay the infinite price of the Passion and death of Christ."[2] This viewpoint reminds us of the graces and gifts received from having to endure the cross of infertility. In prayer, ask God to reveal these to you.

I have been blessed to know people who have seen their infertility as a gift. I cannot say that. However, I can say I have seen gifts come from it. Suffering can become a larger blessing than times of happiness if we view a blessing as any event or thing that brings us closer to God. I have found that my moments of suffering have been the moments when I feel closest to Jesus. Sometimes we fail to see that most of the growth in us has taken place through circumstances we never planned or maybe even wanted, such as infertility.

Monthly Mourning

For me, the feeling of dashed hopes is one of the hardest parts of the process. No matter how many times I tell myself to not grow anxious, as those days when I am supposed to get my period approach, it happens each and every month without fail. There can even be times when I may feel like the journey will never end. I know it is in God's power each and every month, but I struggle with his answer. I try to be hopeful in my waiting, though many times the best I can muster is cautious optimism. It's been hard to undergo this for years, to be told that a certain treatment will solve the problem and get our hopes up only to find the result is the same.

The day my period arrives is often the hardest. The letdown of yet another cycle of disappointment is hard to describe. The temptation to throw myself a pity party is huge. The plans I had right before finding out I got my period change in an instant because now I just feel like wallowing—nothing else seems to matter. It's as if all my energy is zapped in an instant. It's so hard to begin again—to start the process of hoping every month. It is amazing, though, to see the difference a day can make. In my journal, that first day was so filled with sadness, but just the gift of time and perspective can help greatly.

The flip side to the monthly pity party is the temptation to avoid the cross: to be strong, not cry, not grieve, and avoid it all together. God knows how deeply we hurt, and the act of allowing ourselves a day or two of mourning makes the entire process much easier. He wants us to be gentle with ourselves. He knows it is hard to accept the cross, but he challenges us to do so and promises to be there for the journey.

I often find hope in the story of Lazarus's death when Lazarus's sister, Martha, questioned Jesus: "Why didn't you come sooner?" (Jn 11:1–44). There is desperation in Martha's plea that I can relate to. "God, why don't you stop this infertility struggle now? All of this pain wouldn't happen if you would come sooner." The problem with these thoughts, however, is that God is already there. He doesn't need to come; he is there, and for whatever reason, this is happening.

Another way of dealing with a cross is to parcel it out through blame and complaints. There is a temptation at times to regret decisions—to feel like "if only" I would have done something sooner, if only I would have started trying sooner or seen this specialist sooner or taken that medicine or done this test sooner. But all of this fails to take into account how God is in control of everything. We beat ourselves up and don't love ourselves the way he does. We need to remember that God will give us the grace to carry our cross.

We know that time is important for fertility purposes, yet the older we get, the harder it will be to get pregnant. This is hard because society makes it seem like we can study, have a career, and climb the corporate ladder, and when we're done— when we're "ready" (have a house, have traveled, etc.)—then we can get pregnant when we want, but this is not the case. God did not create our bodies this way. I sometimes thought about this since my husband and I postponed pregnancy while I was in graduate school. Should I have gone to school, or should we have simply started having a family right away? However, the guilt and thoughts about wasted time are not beneficial. Even when we started the infertility journey, I can honestly say it was not until over two and a half years after starting that I ever really felt there was a plan in place. We had been seeing doctors and maybe had misplaced loyalty. It was hard not to think about the time that was wasted, all the while thinking how I was getting older and that my mother had menopause early, so I was worried we had lost precious time.

There is sadness every month when no pregnancy is achieved, and no good news is shared with so many friends and family who have walked this journey with us, but each month I choose to keep going, asking God to light our path and guide us to the right place and choices. There is so little we can do. Ultimately, God is the giver and taker of life. All we can do is remain faithful and ask God for the grace to faithfully carry the cross of infertility.

Choosing to See

Choosing to See is the title to a book I read while I was struggling with infertility, and it reminded me of my need to embrace my cross. This book is about a mother's journey through the loss of her daughter. As the author, Mary Beth Chapman, puts it, our faith is either all true or none of it is, and we have to choose to see.[3] Every day that I wake up and have to pull myself together, I can choose to see God's blessings around me or I can choose to look at the pain.

I was recently asked to help plan a baby shower. I can choose to wallow in my own self-pity or self-righteousness, or I can choose to do what I know I am being called to do, which is to help plan the shower and be grateful for the opportunity. In an e-mail response to the person who asked for my help with the shower, I wrote, "Thank you for including me." I honestly had to reread the words because I wanted to make sure they were sincere before I hit "send." I know it's hard to attend baby showers, let alone plan one, but I also know that God's grace will give me the strength to get through anything. This is the spiritual fruit of generosity, which though sour at first, will become sweeter the more I practice it. We are called to use these gifts of the Holy Spirit, and in those moments, when walking into a baby superstore to buy yet another present for someone else, we can avoid a possible breakdown by just stepping away from the situation. Pray, visit the Blessed Sacrament, pick up a prayer book, or pray the Rosary—whatever will get you to focus on God. That first step is the hardest, but you'll be so glad you did. God will meet you more than halfway. He will not force you, though; the choice is yours. Choose to see.

Fighting with Feelings, Doubts, and Fears

Sometimes I struggle with thinking my feelings should be different than they are. After a bad evening recently, my mother told me I don't have to be happy about my infertility, but I do have to accept it. I'm not going to kid God anyway; he knows how I feel. He knows how much it hurts and how much of a sacrifice it is to say, "Your will be done, Lord, not mine." However, I'm often hard on myself for not feeling joyful or happy about my circumstances, but God reminds me that I am human, and my emotions are a part of who I am.

In my humanity, I have struggled with all kinds of ugly feelings: despair, failure, jealousy, anger, hopelessness, bitterness, exhaustion, and resentfulness. At the end of the day, I try to remember that, despite all those feelings, I have never been unloved. There is such power in knowing this and truly internalizing it. Knowing that Jesus loves me regardless of all the horrible things I feel and think motivates me to be better.

One of the most powerful emotions I have experienced during my struggle with infertility is fear. Many times I'm simply afraid of being denied my desire to have more children. I know God knows my heart and the raw emotion I feel, but I grow tired of being told no again and again. I want a different answer, a different outcome. My heart longs to be a mother to more children. As I continue to pray that his will be done in hopes that his will is for us to have more children, I often recall that God tells us to trust in him. "Even the hairs of your head have all been counted. Do not be afraid" (Lk 12:7). I have to choose to have faith. I choose to have faith in God. I choose to know that God knows our deep desire to parent more of his children. I choose to live out the life he has asked us to live, honoring him. It can be scary, but I trust that, if God is taking care of the hairs on my head, he is surely in control of my fertility. As C. S. Lewis is known for saying, "We're not necessarily doubting that God will do the best for us; we are wondering how painful the best will turn out to be." This act of accepting God's will and striving to live joyfully amidst the pain of infertility is how we respond to God's call to "take up one's cross" (Mt 16:24).

Following and Trusting God

Once we have committed to bearing the cross of infertility, we are faced with the challenge of continuing to follow and trust God. This can only happen if we are united with God in prayer and remain hopeful in his plan for us.

The Challenge of Prayer

Wanting a child is something good, and turning to God to express our desire is only natural. With this in mind, how do we reconcile scripture passages such as Matthew 7:7–10?

> Ask and it will be given to you; seek and you will find; knock and the door will be opened to you. For everyone who asks, receives; and the one who seeks, finds; and to the one who knocks, the door will be opened. Which one of you would hand his son a stone when he asks for a loaf of bread, or a snake when he asks for a fish?

Infertility many times made me feel like I was receiving a snake instead of a fish. I rationally know that God understands me more than I understand myself and he knows my needs and my prayers, but when the constant pleas for answers and a cure to our infertility are answered with silence or more questions, it feels like a snake has taken hold of us.

I have chosen to anchor myself in scripture and Catholic theology, and I know that just because I ask for something does not mean I will get it (and thank God for that!), but I also see in scripture many examples of people who kept praying fervently, and I try to use them as an example in my own prayer life. I have always been particularly moved by the parable of the widow and the judge in Luke 18:1–8:

> Then he told them a parable about the necessity for them to pray always without becoming weary. He said, "There was a judge in a certain town who neither feared God nor respected any human being. And a widow in that town used to come to him and say, 'Render a just decision for me against my adversary.' For a long time the judge was unwilling, but eventually he thought, 'While it is true that I neither fear God nor respect any human being, because this widow keeps bothering me I shall deliver a just decision for her lest she finally come and strike me.'" The Lord said, "Pay attention to what the dishonest judge says. Will not God then secure the rights of his chosen ones who call out to him day and night? Will he be slow to answer them? I tell you, he will see to it that justice is done for them speedily. But when the Son of Man comes, will he find faith on earth?"

I know my Father is not a corrupt judge, so I feel that, if a corrupt judge can be moved by the persistence of a widow, my Father may be moved by the pleas of an infertile woman. I know that in the end these pleas are really transforming me and not God. Maybe the mere fact of begging God for children has intensified my prayer life or the knowledge of my complete and total dependence on my Creator for everything.

Prayer has changed me, and I know I need prayer to carry the cross.

I have also learned that we need Mary as our mother to assist in carrying the cross of infertility. My relationship with Mary was never particularly strong growing up, but my faith tells me that she has always interceded for me. The struggle with infertility has led me to turn to her more. I felt that her example of acceptance of God's will was the best example for me, with all the risks she took in saying yes to the Lord. We are called in our infertility to say yes as well—yes to trusting that his will is the only way for us.

I have received reminders of Mary's intercession throughout my journey, most recently in the form of miraculous medals, which I received periodically from the unlikeliest of sources. I find it hard to pray for the miracle of another child, so I pray rather for the miracle of indifference and the miracle of complete trust in the ways of the Lord, as Mary did.

Sometimes I wonder if the changes in my habits and spiritual life because of infertility have been my healing, but since a child is what I desire, I do not realize it. What if I have been healed, but not in the way I have asked for and hence I am like the nine lepers that did not come back to thank Jesus when he miraculously cured them?

There are also examples of people pleading for healing in the Bible:

> And as Jesus passed on from there, two blind men followed [him], crying out, "Son of David, have pity on us!" When he entered the house, the blind men approached him and Jesus said to them, "Do you believe that I can do this?" "Yes, Lord," they said to him. Then he touched their eyes and said, "Let it be done for you according to your faith." And their eyes were opened. (Mt 9:27–30)

So many times I choose to pester God like the widow and the blind men, knowing my Lord doesn't mind my pestering, while trying to accept his will for the answers to my petitions. For me, there have been countless prayers before the Blessed Sacrament, and I have often felt like Hannah, crying my heart out to Jesus only to feel silence or know the answer continues to be, "Wait." In the book of Numbers, the Jewish people express the same sentiments I often feel: "But with their patience worn out by the journey, the people complained against God" (Nm 21:4–5). I, too, am worn out by my journey, and those feelings lead me to complain and whine to God.

But what happens when all you seem to hear in response to your prayers is silence? Though I have been involved in Ignatian retreats for many years and am rather familiar with the silence that is required of a Christian in prayer, I still have found it hard to live in the silence. My heart has many times been restless and grown weary of the silence month after month. It is like being in a desert where I have to depend on him alone. It is possible that the answers lie within the silence, and we get so caught up in our noisy lives that we need to take time to be still. This can be the gift in itself. "Be still and know that I am God" (Ps 46:10).

Sometimes I'm the one who is silent. I sometimes feel so tired, so exhausted, and so utterly done with everything. I don't have any more words, my sighs increase by the day, and I can't seem to muster the smiles I used to in order to hide the pain. Many times when I have come speechless to the Lord, he has heard my heart and given me the gifts I need to continue. "In the same way, the Spirit too comes to the aid of our weakness; for we do not know how to pray as we ought, but the Spirit itself intercedes with inexpressible groanings" (Rom 8:26).

We tend to think of gifts as tangible items wrapped up in boxes and given to us by loved ones, so it can be hard to understand the spiritual gifts that our God is constantly pouring on us. Only through prayer have I really come to understand this. Many times I have prayed, not with the feeling or conviction that I would like, but with the knowledge that my prayer was the correct one—the thing I needed to do.

In so doing, he has given me the peace to react well to certain situations, for example, better than I think I am capable of reacting. I'm not saying this is easy, nor that

> Until you are convinced that prayer is the best use of your time you will not find the time for prayer.
>
> *Fr. Hilary Ottensmeyer, O.S.B.*

I do not have bad days or moments, but I know that God has poured down his Holy Spirit and held onto me as a loving Father, teaching me to rely on him alone throughout this process.

Hoping Beyond Hope

One of the Bible passages I studied and often came back to in prayer is Romans 5:3–5: "More than that, we rejoice in our sufferings, knowing that suffering produces endurance, and endurance produces character, and character produces hope, and hope does not disappoint us, because God's love has been poured into our hearts through the Holy Spirit which has been given to us."

This passage reveals the perseverance required by hope. It is hard to not let difficulties and afflictions get the better of us, but as St. Paul explains, in continuing to build endurance and character, we achieve hope. In *Rain on Me*, the author, Holley Gerth, reflects on this passage and the fact that hope is a process, but in our culture we view hope as an emotion rather than the outcome of choices.[4] It has helped me in my struggle with hope to focus on the process.

The only book of poetry on my nightstand amidst all my books is a collection of poems by Emily Dickinson. It is fitting, then, that one of her most famous poems would deal with something that I have struggled with so deeply during the road of infertility.

Hope

> Hope is the thing with feathers
> That perches in the soul,
> And sings the tune—without the words,
> And never stops at all,
> And sweetest in the gale is heard;
> And sore must be the storm
> That could abash the little bird
> That kept so many warm.
> I've heard it in the chillest land,
> And on the strangest sea;
> Yet, never, in extremity,
> It asked a crumb of me.[5]

I'm from South Florida, which is known for its warm weather and rain. Showers are a regular occurrence, especially in the summer. I try to think of God's grace like that rain, something I can become soaked in, or something I can choose to shield myself from. I need rain, water, and God's grace in order to survive so I know I have to go out there in the storm and weather it to obtain the help I need.

My father's favorite psalm was the popular Psalm 23, which says, "Even when I walk through a dark valley, I fear no harm for you are at my side; your rod and staff give me courage." These words bring me comfort and help me on those days when my hope seems shattered. I feel my earthly and heavenly fathers want these words to give me strength. I pray that you can find strength in these words and in knowing that God is our Good Shepherd who is gently guiding you on the road of infertility.

Prayer to Heal the Pain of Infertility

Dear Lord: The pain of infertility is so deep. All of our lives, we dream of being parents, of raising children with loving hearts to do your will, Lord, on this earth. Month after month when that dream does not come true, it is so painful, Lord. We feel like our dreams die each month with empty arms. Please guide us, Lord, to trust in your plan for us. We desperately need you in our lives. Thank you for all the blessings we do have, knowing through you all things are possible. Amen.[6]

In times of despair and sadness,

- Keep walking—a Chinese proverb says that a journey of a thousand miles begins with just one step. Sometimes that is all we can muster, one step, but that one step is bringing you closer to your destiny.

- Reflect—look back at your journey. Chances are you've come a long way and are stronger now than when you started this journey.

- Call a friend—talking to someone can be a huge help when we are at our lowest. It can be hard to initiate the conversation but it is likely to be worth it.[7]

---

Chapter 7

*B*earing the Cross: A Spirituality of Infertility

The last of the human freedoms is to choose one's
attitude in any given set of circumstances.

Viktor Frankl

Viktor Frankl was an Austrian psychiatrist and neurologist
who survived the Holocaust. While living in a concentration camp, he helped newcomers to the camp deal with their
grief; he believed that one had to fully experience suffering
objectively in order to end it.

Frankl was lucky enough to survive the Nazi concentration camps, but his wife and parents did not. It was due to
his and others' suffering in these camps that he came to the

conclusion that, even in the most painful and challenging situation, life and the suffering therein is meaningful. Frankl recounts an experience he had while working in the harsh conditions of the Auschwitz concentration camp:

> If a prisoner felt that he could no longer endure the realities of camp life, he found a way out in his mental life—an invaluable opportunity to dwell in the spiritual domain, the one that the SS were unable to destroy. Spiritual life strengthened the prisoner, helped him adapt, and thereby improved his chances of survival.[1]

Shortly after his liberation in 1945, Frankl published his best-selling book *Man's Search for Meaning*, which chronicles his experiences as a concentration camp survivor and describes his method of finding meaning in life. The literal translation of the book's original title is "Saying Yes to Life in Spite of Everything: A Psychologist Experiences the Concentration Camp."

It is inspiring and challenging to see that a Holocaust survivor—someone who endured much worse than I ever endured during my walk through infertility—can say "yes to life in spite of everything." Although there were aspects of Frankl's life that were beyond his control while living in the concentration camps, he had a choice about his attitude, and he said yes.

This response is not unlike Mary's *fiat*, of her yes to the Lord in accepting Jesus as her son despite her fear and the risks involved. In the same way, we have a choice about how we will react to the unwelcome guest of infertility—and God wants us to choose to say yes—yes to the cross and yes to all the spiritual lessons that infertility can teach us.

Saying Yes to the Cross

Before Jesus literally took up his own cross, he prayed on the Mount of Olives: "Father, if you are willing, take this cup away from me; still, not my will but yours be done" (Lk 22:42).

So often, I prayed to God to take away the cup of infertility and send us a baby. Unlike Jesus, however, I tended to omit the "not my will but yours be done" part. After all, wasn't my will superior to his?

That veil of self-deception was lifted from my eyes when I started praying St. Ignatius's Principle and Foundation, found in chapter 2. The call to be passionately indifferent is what struck me the most when I first encountered Ignatius's Principle and Foundation while coming to terms with infertility. I was drawn to the invitation to establish order in our lives to enable the transforming love of God to penetrate us.

Being indifferent, then, is having the freedom to constantly love and serve, to go beyond our comfort zones and allow God to weave his will into our lives. A priest I know, Fr. Manuel Maza, S.J., says it's not about making plans and then asking God to conform his plans to ours; it's about praying, "God, give me plans."

Just as it is important to be indifferent in discernment, it is equally important to strive for indifference in our struggle with infertility. Indifference evolves toward openness and commitment. It means putting God's will above all else and seeking to love whatever God wants us to love. It also requires that we not prefer "riches to poverty, honor to dishonor, a long life to a short life" (SE 23). This same concept can be applied to infertility in that God calls us to not prefer sickness to health or infertility to fertility.

To be indifferent to the outcome is not to be indifferent to God's will. To the contrary, it means to be so passionately in love with God that one says yes to his will, even if that means taking up a heavy cross. Being indifferent is a grace from God, and it is necessary to ask God for it. However, saying yes to the cross of infertility is not something that happens overnight, nor do we have to carry this cross alone. We must be patient with ourselves and realize that it is a decision we make daily, with God's help.

I can't say that I ever achieved the complete indifference to which we're called, and I probably didn't relinquish as much control as I would have liked, but prayer did help me surrender a lot (okay, some) of the control to God. Praying for the grace of indifference and making the effort to trust in God's will is a part of the journey of infertility.

It is important to acknowledge the suffering associated with infertility, since one way of managing the pain is to face it. In time we can learn to embrace the cross—otherwise, how do we carry something if we don't fully embrace it? It is so much harder to carry something if we are not putting all of our effort into it. Pray for courage and strength; remember that the Bible tells us not to be afraid 365 times—enough to remind us every day of the year!

As with continuous exercise, carrying our cross helps us build endurance and makes bearing the cross somewhat easier. There are some days when we feel weak and the load doesn't seem so light, but as we accept God's will and grow in his grace, the load doesn't seem as heavy. It may simply be that we become used to carrying it around, but the very act of accepting and carrying the cross helps us on our journey.

Inner Ugliness

Infertility made me feel ugly. I'm not just talking about physically, though, yes, that was part of it, as I ogled at beautiful pregnant bellies and wished I was sporting one, too. What I felt was ugly inside. I had always prided myself on not being an envious person. I was always content with what I had and never coveted what others had; that was until I couldn't have what others had. But I wasn't comfortable with this newfound jealousy. I hated it, actually, and I didn't feel like myself. It was a vicious cycle because the more envy I felt, the worse I felt for feeling that way. I walked around feeling bad for feeling bad.

I was also plagued by my past and felt I was being punished for it. For many years, I did not want to have children and thought that I would make a bad mother. Then I married my husband, a man who was born with a vocation to fatherhood, and that slowly changed. I don't think my fears of parenting ever subsided, though, so when we weren't conceiving as quickly as I would have liked, I felt somewhat justified in doubting my perceived inability to parent and thought God was agreeing with me. I thought I just wasn't a good enough person to be a mother, and in my mind, God seemed to feel the same way, too.

The father of lies has a way of preying on our insecurities and making us believe things that simply aren't true. Don't let evil bully you into thinking that you deserve infertility. I've heard of so many women questioning whether infertility is a punishment from God—for having used birth control, for a past abortion, or for any number of individual reasons—but allow me to set the record straight. God loves me—and *you*— more than we can ever comprehend. He doesn't desire to hurt, tease, or abandon us but rather the contrary.

In fact, God models the loving parent we so long to be. As a Father, he allows us, his children, to fall sometimes so that we may learn to walk. He doesn't ever desire for his children to be harmed, but he also knows that sparing us from heart-breaks and disappointments in life would not help us flourish and grow, nor would we ever realize how dependent on him we really are unless he let us discover that for ourselves.

Even though it must hurt him, God's love for his kids is so great that he has to allow us to experience suffering in life sometimes in order to help us learn and mature, and hope-fully do so with faith. Somehow, in some strange, inexplicable way, infertility is part of his love for us.

Infertility Is a Gift

Hearing that infertility is a gift is about as thrilling as being told to "relax and you'll get pregnant" or "just adopt and you'll be expecting in no time." But the truth is, we have been entrusted with this journey. We have been entrusted by God to grow in patience and to remember that not all things happen when we want them but that all things do "work for good for those who love God, who are called according to his purpose" (Rom 8:28).

One of the foundations of Ignatian spirituality is "finding God in all things." This means that I have to find God in my infertility. It may not be something I want to do at times, but it is something I am called to do. Some people choose to compartmentalize their lives and their religion and keep them separate, but nothing is outside the scope of God. If God is in all things, then the cross of infertility is one that helps me to grow closer to God.

Not everyone is chosen for this cross, but God knows whom he chooses and why. Though we may never know the reasons we were called to experience infertility, it is part of our journey here. As we grow as Christians, we carry our cross with grace and faith in the God who is with us day in and day out at every doctor's appointment, during every failed treatment, for every negative pregnancy test, and for friends' baby showers. Through it all, he carries us and sustains us to keep going and keep trusting.

The Makings of a Miracle

> Little seeds are the almost invisible beginning from which transformation grows. Perhaps part of our problem with miracles is that we try to get at them from the wrong end. We strive to see the end of the miracle—the great transformation, the unexpected cure, or the new life where there was none before. But we very rarely notice the start of the miracle. This is a great pity because, actually, these almost invisible beginnings of the miraculous are all around us. The thing about miracles, of course, is that they usually take time. Perhaps that is the hidden gift of time—the opportunity to grow miracles in it.[2]

Every day as we walk this journey, we await the miracle of a child. But perhaps the miracle is our own transformation into more faithful Christians, Christians who look in awe for miracles all around but find that these miracles start slowly, in the same way that the miracle of a seed becomes a giant tree. Just as a seed needs to be nurtured by sunlight and water in order to grow, we, too, need to nurture ourselves and our relationships with God in order for the miracle of our transformation to transpire.

As Carmen discussed in chapter 6, praying during infertility can be really challenging, but I can't emphasize enough the importance of praying through this process. Though God may at times seem silent, he does listen to us and cradles us in his arms. I had an hour-long commute in each direction to and from work every day, and I would take this time to pray for God to help my husband and me as we longed to expand our family. Whether it be through reading scripture, reading Catholic books, praying the Rosary, practicing personal meditations, or even just crying out to God, prayer is essential to getting us through this difficult time. It is in prayer that God can console us and lead us to his will.

We need to recognize the trial—the transformation—as miraculous and not just look for the end result. Part of my personal transformation while struggling with fertility was that infertility drew me closer to God's Word. One of the passages from scripture that impacted me was Galatians 5:22–23, which says that "the fruit of the Spirit is love, joy, peace, patience, kindness, generosity, faithfulness, gentleness, self-control."

Maybe there is a particular fruit that God needs to cultivate in you. Ask God to show you which fruits need to take root in you and watch as he makes it possible for them to grow.

Infertility in Scripture

Though the apparent rise in infertility cases is recent, infertility has existed since the beginning of time. In the Bible, we are introduced to a number of people who dealt with infertility in their own unique way. By acquainting ourselves with these people, we can find comfort in their stories and recall that we are not alone. These holy men and women who have gone before us know this pain firsthand and clung to God in their most desperate hour.

If we allow God's word to be a lamp for our feet and a light for our path (Ps 119:105), we can join our suffering to that of

Hannah, Sarah, Job, and so many others who struggled to be faithful to God without understanding why they were enduring trials.

> Infertility is part of our faith story. God must hold very dear those who suffer from this pain, for they tend to be the only women in the Bible who are given the special privilege of being named. A pattern will emerge while reading Scripture that shows how God aches over the terrible tragedy of infertility and seeks to bring comfort.[3]

Perhaps it might be beneficial to take one or more of these women as a prayer companion of sorts. In his Spiritual Exercises, "contemplation" is the word St. Ignatius uses to encourage us to "enter a scene" from scripture and allow the Lord to reveal his message to us. Creighton University's Online Ministries offers tips on using all of our senses and imagination to pray with scripture.[4] God can work through our imaginations and can heal us and comfort us. Let's meet these prayer companions now.

Sarah and Abraham

Genesis 16–18, 21

Abraham and Sarah had given up hope of ever having children—so profound was Sarah's despair that she even encouraged Abraham to have relations with her maidservant, Hagar, so that Abraham could have children. God later promised Abraham that he and Sarah would have a son, to which Abraham laughed in disbelief. Sarah had a similar—now infamous—reaction to God's promise. The Lord questioned why Sarah laughed and said, "Is anything too marvelous for the Lord to do? At the appointed time, about this time next year, I will return to you, and Sarah will have a son" (Gn 18:14). Either out of fear or denial, Sarah claimed she hadn't laughed, but the Lord called her bluff.

The Lord kept his promise, and Sarah became pregnant and gave birth to a son, Isaac. Sarah concludes, "God has given me cause to laugh, and all who hear of it will laugh with me. Who would have told Abraham," she added, "that Sarah would nurse children! Yet I have borne him a son in his old age" (Gn 21:6–7).

If all we want to do is laugh at the seemingly fruitless medical interventions or the ridiculous advice that well-meaning people offer to help us conceive, then we're in good company: Sarah and Abraham laughed, too. Or maybe we've gotten to the point in our infertility journey where we, like Sarah, feel it is impossible for God to give us a child, and the thought of having one at this point seems almost humorous. In Sarah, we find that we can even laugh at God over the whole journey of infertility and its sometimes unexpected results. God's ways are not our ways, and sometimes we're the ones laughing; other times, God gets the last laugh. Despite our incredulity, we must remember that the word "impossible" is not in God's vocabulary. All things are possible for him.

Isaac and Rebekah
Genesis 25:19–24

Abraham and Sarah's son, Isaac, married Rebekah when he was forty years old. Isaac prayed to the Lord on behalf of Rebekah, who was sterile, and after twenty years of marriage, the Lord blessed them with twin boys, Esau and Jacob.

If someone in our family has been unable to conceive, do we fear that may be our plight, too? Isaac and Rebekah faced infertility just as Abraham and Sarah had, and perhaps they were concerned, too. Our family history may be a concern for us, but the Great Physician treats us each as individual patients and covers us with the healing salve of his love.

Jacob and Rachel
Genesis 29:30–30:24

Jacob, son of Isaac and Rebekah, married sisters Rachel and Leah. Leah and Jacob had six sons and a daughter, but the Lord had closed Rachel's womb. Rachel tried everything she could think of to have children, even claiming as her own two children that Jacob conceived with her maidservant. Once in anguish, she cried out to Jacob, "Give me children, or I shall die" (Gn 30:1). It wasn't until the Lord opened her womb many years later that she bore two sons, Joseph and Benjamin.

The story of Rachel is very powerful because she best demonstrates the anguish that those experiencing infertility sometimes struggle with. In times of great despair, we can ask Rachel to intercede for us.

Rachel also knows the pain of jealousy—her own sister had seven children with Isaac during the time that she remained barren. They say time heals all wounds, but as is often the case in infertility, the passage of time only serves to heighten the sense of despair and envy, and this was indeed the case for Rachel, who expressed her anger and frustration with Jacob and with God.

We need to be prayerfully introspective and honest with our feelings during this difficult walk. Whatever it is we feel, God can handle it! In the case of potentially sinful attitudes such as envy, however, we need to ask God to help heal us and change our hearts. We can also ask for his forgiveness in the Sacrament of Reconciliation. We don't solve anything by remaining angry or envious. In the end, as with Rachel, it is up to the Lord and his perfect timing, his *kairos*, to determine when this journey will end.

Hannah

I Samuel I

Elkanah had two wives, his favorite of which was Hannah. His other wife, Peninnah, taunted Hannah for being barren, at which point Hannah would weep and refuse to eat.

Once, while the family made a pilgrimage to the temple, Hannah, "in her bitterness, prayed to the Lord, weeping copiously" (1 Sm 1:10.) Hannah pleaded with God for a son, promising to give him back in service of the Lord. Eli, seeing her in the temple crying and praying, accused her of being drunk. Hannah explained that she was simply "an unhappy woman" who was "only pouring out my troubles to the Lord" and that her prayer was prompted by "deep sorrow and misery" (1 Sm 1:15–16). God answered her prayer with the birth of Samuel, the last and greatest judge of Israel.

Hannah just might be the Biblical poster child for infertile women. Just look at all the words used to describe how Hannah felt: bitterness, weeping copiously, unhappy, deep sorrow, and misery. Do these feelings sound familiar? Despite how sad she was, these feelings did not impede Hannah from praying fervently and pouring out her troubles to the Lord. It didn't matter to her if she looked like a drunk; she was not afraid of asking God for her most ardent desire to bear a child. Sometimes we may face criticism by others (as Hannah endured at the hands of Peninnah) for how we're handling infertility or for what treatments we choose to pursue (or not pursue). We're called not to focus on what others think but instead, like Hannah, to keep our eyes on God.

It is also interesting to note that, after she prayed intensely, she returned to her husband and "no longer appeared downcast" (1 Sm 1:18). This is what prayer does: it doesn't always change our situation; it changes our outlook. Time spent praying before the Blessed Sacrament, the Catholic answer to Hannah's temple pilgrimage, is invaluable for changing our perspective on infertility, and we challenge you to spend some time regularly before Christ as you bear the cross of infertility. In Christ's presence at the Blessed Sacrament, we can gaze at him gazing at us and loving us as we are. We can also pour out our troubles to the Lord, as Hannah did, and know we have a captive audience in Jesus.

Zechariah and Elizabeth
Luke 1:5–25, 36–37, 57–58

Elizabeth and Zechariah were "righteous in the eyes of God, observing all the commandments and ordinances of the

Lord blamelessly, but they had no child" because Elizabeth was barren and they were both advanced in years (Lk 1:6–7). That scripture even makes reference to the fact that they were good people but hadn't conceived reminds us that, despite what may have been portrayed historically (or any insecurities we ourselves may have), infertility is not a punishment or a curse.

Though they figured they would never have a child given their age, an angel appeared to Zechariah and promised them a son, John the Baptist, who prepared the way for Jesus. When Elizabeth found out they had conceived, she expressed her faithfulness and trust in God's timing: "So has the Lord done for me at a time when he has seen fit to take away my disgrace before others" (Lk 1:25). We often think we know the best time for us to have children, but we can sometimes forget that we receive children from God in his time, not ours.

Elizabeth also mentions the "disgrace" of infertility. It is challenging sometimes, in Catholic circles especially, to be the only family without children or to have a comparatively small family. Inappropriate questions and comments do not help the situation.

But God doesn't want to embarrass or disgrace us. When the angel Gabriel appeared to Mary at the annunciation, he told her that Elizabeth had also conceived a son and reminded her—and us as well—that "nothing is impossible for God" (Lk 1:37). Just as he had with Sarah, God made the impossible possible. How big is our faith, and how deep is our hope? Do we limit God's power and protect ourselves from getting hurt by assuming he can't do what to us seems impossible? And what is it that we assume he can't do? Perhaps what we think is impossible God has already made possible, but we haven't asked God what his plans are for how that will transpire—and it may look completely different from what we planned. Just ask Zechariah and Elizabeth, and all the other couples who faced infertility in the Bible.

A Journey to God

Each of the couples in scripture who faced infertility dealt with it in different ways and exhibited different spiritualities. Abraham and Sarah were incredulous. Rachel was anguished but honest. Hannah was persistent and prayerful. Zechariah was speechless (literally). Elizabeth was trusting and faithful.

In the same way, we each approach the Lord in different ways during our infertility journey, whether broken or hopeful. Each person's path is different, but the point of the journey is to get closer not just to a baby but more importantly to God. By definition, spirituality is a way of relating to God, and infertility makes you find your own way of relating to God. Although it is *not* in our control to ensure the journey will bear fruit in our wombs, it *is* up to us to ensure that this path will bear spiritual fruit.

Help! I Need Somebody

In addition to the holy examples from scripture whom we can ask to pray for us, there also are saints that our faith has associated with infertility. Just as we would ask a friend to pray for us, we can ask St. Gerard Majella, Sts. Anne and Joachim (Mary's parents and Jesus' grandparents), and St. Gianna Beretta Molla for their intercession and prayers to help us through infertility. St. Anthony and St. Rita of Cascia are also saints associated with infertility. If words fail you, see the end of the chapter for more information on these saints, and find prayers for their intercession throughout the book at the closing of each chapter.

Even when these holy men and women and their stories are of help to us, sometimes we just long to have a friend in the flesh who will listen to us vent, empathize with what we're feeling, and hand us a hankie when the tears start to flow. So where do Catholics experiencing infertility go for help and support?

The online Catholic infertility blog community has become a huge source of support. Starting around 2006, a number of Catholic women have been blogging (online journaling) about their experiences with infertility.[5] The blogs chronicle their emotions, their treatments (many using NaPro-TECHNOLOGY), and in some cases, their good news when pregnancy has occurred. What started as women from different parts of the nation chronicling their individual journeys has become an online support system where they comment and offer prayers on one another's blogs. Some have even met in person. We estimate there are at least forty blogs written by Catholic women currently experiencing infertility or who have walked the pain of infertility and now have a child. Anyone is welcome to read and comment on the blogs, and women often find a kinship and a depth of understanding on these Web pages that they aren't finding elsewhere. See a list of just some of these blogs at the end of the chapter. You may even find that starting your own blog to transcribe your thoughts during infertility may be cathartic and healing.

One of these bloggers also started an infertility support group called Sarah-Hannah-Elizabeth (SHE), which meets monthly in Kentucky for prayer and discussion. A support group called Hannah's Heart was started in Jacksonville, Florida. Other infertility support ministries are offered by Elizabeth Ministry or pro-life ministries. Check your parish and diocese to see if there are any support groups in your area. If not, gather a group of friends to pray along with the infertile couples from scripture and discuss what their stories mean to you. In addition to helping you air out your emotions, these groups can help you grow in grace when they are centered on God.

The support doesn't always have to come from people experiencing infertility. Carmen was one of my biggest sources of encouragement, empathy, and support while my husband and I were walking through infertility, and this was years before she experienced it herself. Meeting with a Catholic counselor or spiritual director may also be necessary and helpful in this journey. This can come by way of a psychologist or therapist who shares your faith and values or a priest or religious. There is no shame in this—Carmen and I have each met with a Catholic psychologist through the years and have found it extremely helpful and edifying.

Sing a New Song

I became so weary with myself during this journey that I had to find new and creative ways to overcome my pessimism. So I created a CD of uplifting songs, both contemporary religious and motivational secular songs, to help me while lamenting not having a child. I would listen to the CD, which I titled "Songs of Hope," on my commute to help me stay positive and focus on God. Consider creating a playlist for yourself that helps remind you of God's love and hope.

Focusing on God and trying to keep positive, even amidst the suffering, can help us change the burden of infertility into a blessing: "Sing to the Lord a new song; sing to the Lord, all the earth. Sing to the Lord, bless his name; proclaim his salvation day after day. Tell his glory among the nations; among all peoples, his marvelous deeds" (Ps 96:1–3).

Prayer for the Intercession of St. Mary and St. Elizabeth

Wonderful Lord, as we read about Mary's visit with Elizabeth, we are reminded that You are a God of joy and that You always fulfill Your promises. We ask the Blessed Mother to intercede for us when we feel discouraged, so that our souls may always magnify You, O Lord. May she remind us of Your promises and Your faithfulness when the difficulties of life cover us with darkness. Give us spirits that rejoice in You, our Savior, for all the great things that you have done for us and will continue to bestow upon us, simply because You love us.

We also ask for the intercession of St. Elizabeth, whose child leaped with joy within her at the presence of Mary and the Blessed Jesus within her womb. May we also leap for joy in knowing that they are always present with us, too. Give us the patience and hope of Elizabeth during the barren times of our lives, so that we may trust and pray with confidence in God's eternal promises for us.

Blessed Mary and Elizabeth, pray for us.

Further Reading

There are a myriad of Catholic blogs dedicated to the infertility journey. Some have conceived or have adopted since starting their infertility blog; others are still waiting to become parents. It is impossible to list them all, but here is a sampling; some of these blogs have links to other infertility blogs on their site:

All You Who Hope:
http://allyouwhohope.blogspot.com

A Martha Trying to Be Mary:
http://amarthatryingtobemary.blogspot.com

The Apostolate of Hannah's Tears:
http://theapostolateofhannahstears.blogspot.com

Frustrated Musings of a Seemingly Calm Gal:
http://frustrationstation-jellybelly.blogspot.com

Grace in My Heart:
http://graceinmyheart.blogspot.com

Joy Beyond the Cross:
http://joybeyondthecross.blogspot.com

Matching Moonheads:
http://matchingmoonheads.wordpress.com

Pray, Hope, Don't Worry:
http://rhiannon1980.blogspot.com

This Cross I Embrace:
http://thiscrossiembrace.blogspot.com

If you consider joining the infertility online community, here are some commonly used acronyms and abbreviations:

2WW—two-week wait
AF—"Aunt Flo" or another term for getting your period

BBT—basal body temperature
BD—baby dance (sex)
CD—cycle day
CM—cervical mucus
CrM—Creighton method
DH—dear husband
Endo—endometriosis
EW—egg white (in reference to fertile-type mucus)
GIFT—gamete intrafallopian transfer
HSG—hysterosalpingogram (medical test to check fallopian tubes)
M/C—miscarriage
OPK—ovulation predictor kit
PCOS—polycystic ovarian syndrome
PP6 or PPVI—Pope Paul VI Institute in Omaha
RE—reproductive endocrinologist
SA—semen analysis
TCM—traditional Chinese medicine
TTC—trying to conceive

Patron Saints of Infertility

St. Gerard Majella—Although not officially recognized by the Church as such, Catholics have long prayed to this Redemptorist priest as the protector of expectant mothers and the infertile. It is said that St. Gerard was leaving a family he went to visit and dropped his handkerchief. A young woman picked it up and went to give it to him. He told her to keep it, that it would be useful to her in the future. Years later, the young lady was in labor and was dying. She asked for the handkerchief and held it to her womb. Her pain immediately stopped, and she delivered a healthy baby.

St. Gianna Beretta Molla—An Italian mother of four and physician who heroically refused potentially life-saving medical treatment during her last pregnancy in order to save her unborn child. She is a modern-day example of virtue that has been linked to the pro-life movement and motherhood.[6]

St. Anne and Joachim—An ancient story dating to the first centuries of the Church's life recalls how Saints Anne & Joachim [parents of Mary], like Abraham and Sarah, were scorned by their neighbors because they had no children.

"Years of longing did not weaken their trust in God, but grief eventually drove Saint Joachim into the wilderness to fast and pray. Saint Anne, remaining at home, dressed in mourning clothes and wept because she had no child of her own. Seeing her mistress distressed, a servant girl reminded Anne to put her trust in God. Saint Anne washed her face, put on her bridal clothes and went to a garden to plead with God for a child.

"Angels appeared to Saint Anne in her garden and Saint Joachim in the desert, promising that, despite their old age, they would give birth to a child who would be known throughout the world. The new parents ran to meet one another at Jerusalem's Golden Gate, and with a kiss rejoiced in the new life which God had promised would be theirs. Saints Anne and Joachim are powerful intercessors for all married couples, expectant mothers and married couples who are having difficulty conceiving, as well as all who have grown old."[7]

Shrines

St. Lucy's Church—National Shrine of St. Gerard
118 7th Ave., Newark, NJ 07104
(973) 803-4200
www.saintlucy.net/home.html

Our Lady of La Leche Shrine
27 Ocean Avenue, St. Augustine, FL 32084
(904) 824-2809 or (800) 342-6529
www.missionandshrine.org/la_leche.htm

Prayer to Our Lady of La Leche

L ovely Lady of La Leche, most loving Mother of the Child Jesus, and my mother, listen to my humble prayer. Your motherly heart knows my every wish, my every need. To you only, his spotless Virgin Mother, has your Divine Son given to understand the sentiments which fill my soul. Yours was the sacred privilege of being the Mother of the Savior. Intercede with him now, my loving mother, that, in accordance with

his will, I may become the mother of other children of our
heavenly Father. This I ask, O Lady of La Leche, in the name
of your Divine Son, My Lord and Redeemer. Amen.[8]

Resources

Catholic Infertility Support Yahoo! Group:
http://health.groups.yahoo.com/group/catholic-fertility

Elizabeth Ministry:
www.elizabethministry.com

Hannah's Heart Catholic Infertility Support Group:
www.hannahsheart.org

Marie Meaney, *Embracing the Cross of Infertility*, Front Royal/
VA: HLI, 2010.

The St. Gerard Store (handkerchiefs and other items for purchase): www.thesaintgerardstore.com/orderform.html

SHE (Sarah-Hannah-Elizabeth) Infertility Support Group:
www.shesupportgroup.blogspot.com

$\mathcal{I}$nfertility's Effect on Marriage

When we are at peace, we find the freedom to be most fully who we are, even in the worst of times. We let go of what is nonessential and embrace what is essential. We empty ourselves so that God may more fully work within us. And we become instruments in the hands of the Lord.

Joseph Cardinal Bernardin

The rocky road of infertility can have a tremendous impact on a couple's marriage. It can be a time of struggle or a time of growth—or both—depending on how the couple approaches this cross. Within this larger (albeit heavier) cross of infertility are lots of little crosses along the way that will try the couple's relationship. However, there are steps couples can take to ensure that their infertility journey strengthens their marriage.

Crucifix Above the Marriage Bed

Hanging a crucifix above the bed is a very Catholic custom; it's also a very relevant custom for couples that are open to life and God's will for their family. The image of Christ crucified reminds us that the very place where new life is supposed to be created can be the source of the greatest suffering. The same can be said of the marriage bed.

My husband and I did not have a crucifix over our bed when we got married, and while we were struggling with infertility, I asked for this sacramental as an anniversary gift. I wanted a crucifix, not a simple cross, and I was very explicit about this. As children, we often turn away from Jesus on the crucifix, but as adults, we realize that life is precisely about dying—dying to self.

The wisdom in having a crucifix over the marriage bed is that we are to die to ourselves to some degree during the marital act and die to the outcome of our relations. The crucifix has also helped me to keep focus and keep working on our marriage. There are times when the fruitlessness of our lovemaking seemingly tarnishes the act itself, but seeing Christ crucified and uniting our suffering to him helps us to gain perspective.

St. John Chrysostom is known for teaching that the marriage bed is one of the four altars in our home, and it's important to maintain that altar as a sacred space. This means no TVs, no computers, and no phones—no distractions—have your bedroom be a sanctuary. Do we bring cell phones and laptops into Church with us to use them while the sacrifice of the Mass is transpiring on the altar before us? Of course not—to do this would be to defile the sacred altar of Christ. In the same way, bringing distractions into the bedroom detracts from the sacredness of the marital altar and the self-sacrifice and love that takes place upon it.

During a period of time while we were struggling with infertility I would bring more distractions into the bedroom than before, maybe subconsciously to not have to deal with certain emotions. As I reflected on the words of St. John Chrysostom, I knew I needed to stop using the laptop in the room, stop watching TV, and just focus on our bedroom as a sanctuary, a place of retreat from the rest of the world.

Intimacy

Intimacy can be greatly affected by infertility. For example, with prescribed abstinence and scheduled intimacy, spontaneity is lost. So often, I felt that the "fun" of having a baby disappeared along the way. I distinctly remember my husband telling others how great it was to try to have a baby. We went from years of practicing Natural Family Planning (NFP), postponing a pregnancy while I finished graduate studies, to having the freedom of complete openness to God's plan. However, this all changes when there are doctors telling us how and when to make love. For some, this can make marital relations feel like a chore or another task to add to an endless to-do list. In our constant illusion that we have more control than we do, it also places tons of pressure on whether we get our timing wrong or we miss our window instead of enjoying the gift of our sexuality.

Problems infertility can have on marriage:

- Seeking to create life may cause death of marriage
- Disappointment and shame of such a public cross
- High divorce rates
- Reproductive problems are often not anticipated, and there is a lot of anger (taking for granted that couples can have kids when they decide to)
- Suffering in silence
- Both a physical and a psychological problem—often only the first part is addressed

In our case, because Alex was found to be "subfertile," we had required abstinence leading up to ovulation. This created a strain on our marriage and a frustration on both our parts. Waiting until happy faces showed up on ovulation predictors was not a happy time for us. Added to that was a self-imposed pressure that we had to make love on certain days to not miss an opportunity.

A friend who struggled with infertility for many years told me that sexual relations were something she and her husband did not even think about because the doctors were so involved they dictated what went on with her and her husband. We need to be very careful to not allow this type of invasion of our bedroom to occur.

Recalling both the unitive and procreative elements of conjugal love, it is critically important to have sex even when there is no baby to be had. Sex helps men relax and feel loved. Conversely, women need to feel loved in order to relax and have sex, but we need to make an effort in this area so that our sexual union does not revolve solely around having a child. It may be easier said than done, but pray and ask God for the grace to overcome these preoccupations.

Being There

During our struggle with infertility, my husband and I went to a Steven Curtis Chapman concert, a contemporary Christian musician who is easily my favorite artist. He is the author of our wedding song, which we have had the privilege to hear live quite a few times now. The words of our wedding song, "I Will Be Here," have exemplified our time of infertility. When we chose the song, I could not have known how powerful the words would be. Infertility makes it seem like the sun does not appear, and we lose sight of love easily, but the song's chorus is so simple yet so poignant: "I will be here." The song doesn't talk about anything other than just being there, but our mere presence is incredibly important to our spouse. We don't always have the perfect words to say to one another and may not know what to do, but we can be there for each other, and that can make all the difference.

Living Our Marriage Vows

When we said the famous "in sickness and in health" vow on our wedding day, most of us were probably not thinking about infertility (at least I know I wasn't). Yet so many couples have come to experience this illness so profoundly in their marriage.

In chapter 2, we discussed the marriage vow as *receiving* children from the Lord and how we did not fully understand that commitment the day we made it. Another vow that has taken on new meaning on this infertility journey is "I will love you and honor you all the days of my life." Honoring our spouses is extremely important in all of marriage. In the case of infertility, each spouse may be willing to undergo different treatments, or one may be ready to move on to another option such as adoption. This can be very difficult and requires a great deal of prayer. We have known many couples who differed on the decision to pursue adoption. From my own experience (and it has also happened to other friends), sometimes you simply have to trust the Holy Spirit and his guidance for your spouse. God guides us in ways we do not understand, but his presence is there. It is important to honor, trust, and respect one other during this process.

Do not rush into decisions, and even if you are willing to adopt and your spouse is not, you should not press, but pray. If this is the calling for your family, your spouse will get there eventually, and God will guide you both.

I have struggled greatly in this area, but I have come to realize I am called to recognize Christ in my husband and allow him to take the spiritual lead of the family, in the same way that he would sacrifice himself for me as Jesus has. The following excerpt from scripture has helped me realize this:

> Be subordinate to one another out of reverence for Christ. Wives should be subordinate to their husbands as to the Lord. For the husband is head of his wife just as Christ is head of the church, he himself the savior of the body. As the church is subordinate to Christ, so wives should be subordinate to their husbands in everything. Husbands, love your wives, even as Christ loved the church and handed himself over for her to sanctify her, cleansing her by the bath of water with the word, that he might present

> to himself the church in splendor, without spot or wrinkle
> or any such thing, that she might be holy and without
> blemish. So [also] husbands should love their wives as
> their own bodies. He who loves his wife loves himself.
> For no one hates his own flesh but rather nourishes and
> cherishes it, even as Christ does the church, because we
> are members of his body. "For this reason a man shall
> leave [his] father and [his] mother and be joined to his
> wife, and the two shall become one flesh." (Eph 5:21–31)

I have often said to others that I know the grace that
flowed from the sacrament we entered into on June 16, 2001,
is what has held us together in our marriage. This grace is
very real and allows us to be Christ for our spouse. The grace
that is received from the sacrament of marriage also has been
instrumental in getting us through all that has come our way,
including infertility. Sacramental marriage transforms love.
These vows can serve as a guiding light for us on our journey.
They create the covenant with our spouse and can even help
us in making decisions regarding our infertility. Infertility has
made me realize how only through Christ can we fully live
up to the call of marriage.

Different Places

Difficulty arises when we find ourselves at a different
point in the journey than our spouse. For example, our spouse
may be interested in pursuing treatments that are not in line
with Church teaching. What can we do in these situations?
We need to first of all remember that sin is never an option;
we can only discern between two goods. If our spouse wants
to pursue further treatment that we are not comfortable with,
we need to talk honestly to our spouse about our concerns.
Love is only real and true when it is freely given, and for this
reason we cannot force our spouse to do something against
his or her will—and he or she should not pressure us into
harming our soul. This may be difficult for some spouses to
accept, especially those who differ in spiritual maturity, but

it is critical that we respect one another's consciences and not succumb to pressures to abandon our values.

Seeking the counsel of a good Catholic psychologist, priest, or religious can be very helpful in this situation since it may be easier for a third party to challenge both spouses with understanding one another while remaining faithful to Church teaching. It is also very important that the "why" of the Church's teachings be explained well to a spouse who is questioning the Church's position. Hopefully, through an understanding of the love with which the Church teaches us, both spouses will have a greater capacity to love one another and remain faithful to Christ. A great deal of prayer, love, communication, respect, and gentleness are needed to help overcome this obstacle of differing views on licit treatment. We cannot underestimate the importance of praying for our spouses.

Sometimes it may not involve illicit treatment but simply a different place in formation. We have known several friends who arrived at the decision to adopt at a different time than their spouse. It is important not only to challenge our spouse when necessary but also to lovingly accept that God is working with each of us in a different way and possibly at a different pace.

Facing Gender Differences

Men and women deal with obstacles differently, and this dynamic can be one that affects the marital relationship as well. Chapter 9, which addresses the male perspective on infertility, will go into greater detail on this topic. Essentially, God created us to complement each other. Women, for example, tend to work through their problems by talking about things. Men, on the other hand, often need time and space to process things. My husband would frequently tell me that he did not want to talk about how he was feeling because that would not "solve anything." I had to learn to respect that.

Also, men sometimes feel the need to try to "fix" the situations that their wives may be telling them about, but wives often do not want solutions; they only want to be heard. Because God in his infinite wisdom made us complementary, we need to work at recognizing these gender differences and working through them. As a woman, I had to learn to give my husband the space he needed to process his emotions and also to learn to bite my tongue on many occasions. My husband also learned to listen without offering solutions unless requested. These changes required effort on both our parts, but they helped us solidify the fact that we were in this together.

Equally Painful

Pain has a way of making us focus on ourselves and maybe forget to think of our spouse. If one person has the medical "problem," you have to accept them with their infertility. The temptation to blame the other is especially great and dangerous when only one of you seemingly has a medical condition, but as St. Paul tells us, "the two shall become one flesh" through the sacrament of marriage. It is no longer just one spouse who may have an issue; the couple is infertile, and both spouses, together, must walk this road. For this reason, it's important to realize that pain is shared by both spouses.

In Genesis 30:1–2, we see an envious Rachel tell Jacob, "Give me children or I shall die!" When I read these words in scripture, I can feel the anger, the desperation, and frustration that lead to the bitterness Rachel exhibits. It can be easy to blame the other person as Rachel does. "In anger Jacob retorted, 'Can I take the place of God, who has denied you the fruit of the womb?'" Jacob's words are not only strong but also fundamentally true; we need to remember that God is God and we are not. Rachel goes on to be the mother of Joseph (of *Technicolor* fame) who saved the Israelites from famine. In God's merciful love for us, he has allowed us to suffer infertility. We should not take out our frustration on our spouse.

Additionally, one spouse may seemingly be dealing with infertility just fine while the other is suffering more. We should remember that no one knows the depths of another's heart, and often one spouse may be more in touch with those feelings than the other. It can be frustrating to feel disconnected and in greater pain, but it doesn't mean the other spouse isn't being affected. It is important to discuss this openly and to be patient with one another and each individual's particular way of processing things.

Infertility has made both of us reach beyond what we thought we could, and we have done so together. My husband takes a great deal of pride in being super healthy and not getting sick. After his diagnosis, it took him close to one year to decide to undergo surgery, but as I sat by his bedside at the hospital I knew how much he had sacrificed for us, for our family. He did what he could to improve our chances of getting pregnant. We both did all we could licitly do, enduring physical pain and discomfort in order to help us reach our goal. We did all we could—all the tests and recommended procedures—and then knew all that was left was to continue trusting in God.

Pray as a Couple

A mentor couple in our parish shared with us many years ago that they pray before making love. At first, I honestly found this very strange and was not interested in implementing this into our married life. With infertility, though, came the increased awareness and need for God as the creator of new life. Alex and I began doing this, not as an amulet or something that we thought "if we do this, we'll get pregnant," but really praying that we recognized God's presence in this area of our relationship. I think it has been healing for us to pray in this way.

In Tobit 8:4–8, we find a beautiful example of this same practice that I hope can be of help:

> Tobiah arose from bed and said to his wife, "My love, get up. Let us pray and beg our Lord to have mercy on us and to grant us deliverance."

She got up, and they started to pray and beg that deliverance might be theirs. He began with these words: "Blessed are you, O God of our fathers; praised be your name forever and ever. Let the heavens and all your creation praise you forever.

"You made Adam and you gave him his wife Eve to be his help and support; and from these two the human race descended. You said, 'It is not good for the man to be alone; let us make him a partner like himself.' Now, Lord, you know that I take this wife of mine not because of lust, but for a noble purpose. Call down your mercy on me and on her, and allow us to live together to a happy old age." They said together, "Amen, amen."

Communication

Sometimes infertility can feel isolating even though you are going through it together with your spouse. As such, it's important to make an even greater effort at communication and to talk more about each others' feelings and the situation.

Communication during all of marriage is extremely important, but we must also make an extra effort to communicate with our spouse regarding infertility. We may think that our spouse knows how we are feeling because he or she is the other person most affected by this, but we need to vocalize our thoughts and share so that we truly can be helpmates to each other.

It is amazing how our spouse, the one person who best understands the difficulty of infertility, is often the one from whom we grow distant. In my marriage, it was sometimes frustrating to try to talk to my husband about treatments and to get feedback but instead end up explaining a bunch of things that I felt he should have known. I needed to be more patient with him. I was normally the one contacting doctors and doing research so of course I knew more, and for him, the long list of doctors, medications, and opinions was overwhelming. I know rationally why he needed me to clarify so often, but I would grow inpatient with him because I felt that, in my having to clarify, it was as if he didn't care enough to have remembered originally. Going to each other's doctors' appointments can help you both stay informed and be supportive of each other. It can be difficult to take time off of work to go, but just knowing that the other is there physically can be so important.

Some appointments and procedures are more difficult than others, so if time off of work is an issue, prioritizing and discussing which ones your spouse wants you present for is a good idea. There was a day when I had to see my obstetrician to check how I was responding to a treatment, and while in the waiting room I overheard multiple women discuss their unplanned pregnancies and how they did not want any more children. This was in addition to the parade of bellies on display as I waited. It was hard to be there, but I remember how much better I felt after my husband arrived. It was a routine exam, one I had done several times before, but knowing we were in this together made all the difference for me that day.

All too often, we speak before thinking. One incident relating to infertility (because there are so many outside this area as well!) includes a time that I asked my husband to get me a glass of water after I had already put in a prescribed vaginal progesterone suppository. He told me I should get it myself. Had he thought about it before speaking, he would have realized that I could not get up without risking the suppository coming out before it had a chance to start absorbing.

To his credit, my husband has been extremely supportive of me with this same progesterone treatment. It was recommended that I prop my legs up for one hour after placing the suppository, and Alex very graciously places pillows under my legs and covers me with a blanket while I lie there. It may not seem like a big deal, but through that small act, he shows his support for me.

Team Players

My husband is a huge sports fan, and baseball is his favorite. He always tells people that he knew he had found the right woman when I agreed to go to an Oakland A's baseball game on our honeymoon. One of the aspects of sports that Alex loves is that all the players work together for a common goal. Infertility requires a team as well. The husband and wife are the co-captains of the team, and staying connected to one another requires a lot of teamwork, including communicating effectively and realizing that you need each other in order to succeed.

The infertility team will have other players as well—the doctors you choose, your cheerleaders (family, friends, and support people), and so forth. You and your husband have to draft people with caution. Think about whom you want to share the news of your infertility with. You may want to tell some people so they can give you your space and not pressure you as a couple, or you may want to keep it private, telling only essential people.

Protect Your Marriage Prayerfully

Alex and I were involved in marriage ministry before we realized our infertility. The first few years of our marriage proved to be rather difficult (thank God for sacramental grace), and we fought to improve our relationship. We sought out the help of a Catholic psychologist and have continued to meet with him as needed. It can be difficult to seek the help we may need because pride may get in the way. I'm not going to say it is easy to see someone and share our failings, but in a similar way to confession or spiritual direction, it is important for our spiritual growth.

It is especially important to find a therapist who shares our same beliefs and values and is not going to steer us wrong with his or her advice. We have had friends go to counseling with whoever was on their insurance's list and were told some pretty outlandish things that ultimately hurt their marriages.

As Psalm 25:14 says, "The counsel of the Lord belongs to the faithful; the covenant instructs them."

We also recommend joining a couples group at your parish and becoming involved in marriage ministry. We are involved with marriage preparation in our archdiocese as well as with a marriage movement, and we have found this focus on service has been a huge blessing and source of strength. We served on several retreats during this time and attended a few to enrich our marriage.

The Spiritual Exercises of St. Ignatius of Loyola, which are very powerful silent retreats, can be especially helpful for all of the crossroads we face on this journey, especially in helping us discern what God is calling us to do along the road of infertility. Consider attending a marriage encounter or another retreat that gives you tools to build up your marriage. There are also many resources that can help us online, such as the United States Conference of Catholic Bishops' (USCCB) For Your Marriage initiative.[1]

Service Is Joy

The Indian poet Rabindranath Tagore is cited as the source of the old adage "I slept and dreamt that life was joy. I awoke and saw that life was service. I acted and behold, service was joy." These words are simple, but the message is profound: life is about service, and in that, there is joy. One of our callings as Christians is to serve. Service isn't always easy, but it is necessary for the growth of one's marriage. Psychologists often suggest that those who struggle with depression involve themselves in a form of community service or another means of helping other people. Serving the Lord as a couple can be a means for healing in one's marriage, or it can be a way to bond when you begin to feel distant. Our Church offers us endless possibilities for service according to whatever charism and gifts we have received, and we need to remember that, while we wait, we can put these gifts to use for God's kingdom.

The second letter from St. Paul to Timothy reminds us that we are running the race while we wait, which from an imagery point of view seems odd, but we need to keep moving despite the waiting that is occurring in this area of our lives. We cannot stop serving God; we cannot stop worshipping.

Friends and Our Marriage

It's also important to have friends who can support you in your marriage as you struggle with infertility. My husband and I have been very blessed in this way. God has put holy people in our path who are also trying to live out their vocation of marriage in the best way they can. Some of these friends have experienced infertility and some have not, but all of them support us and pray for us. They listen to us and provide a sounding board for our concerns.

Some of our friends who have experienced infertility have also been examples to us as we journey behind them on this road. They help us navigate the crazy and confusing world of infertility by offering their wisdom and perspective. These couples were great resources for us, both in terms of practical tips like recommending doctors and adoption agencies and most importantly in providing spiritual support. We knew these friends were praying for us and that they were also there for us.

Other couples we spoke to also reiterated the importance of a faith community to sustain them during this difficult time. If you do not have these types of friendships currently, perhaps joining a ministry for couples experiencing infertility may be a place to build these bonds. If this type of group does not exist in your area, God may be challenging you to start one. The Elizabeth Ministry is another ministry that can be helpful and enriching.[2] Perhaps in your parish or through your service you can find the friendships that will help your marriage.

However, we need to remember to keep our marriage sacred and not let outside influences take on too much importance. Within our circle of friends also experiencing infertility, we saw the end of a marriage because of the involvement of outside influences. This couple grew apart after years of marriage, and the rift led to infidelity. We need to remember that other couples can be helpful as long as they are good influences.

As I watched others begin to struggle in their marriages, I wondered how much the heartbreak of this cross impacted these spouses who grew apart. Several friends also shared how infertility was the darkest point in their marriage, and they almost divorced because of the struggle. It is important to remember that God has chosen you to carry this cross together, and the journey, though challenging, can be a great strength to your marriage. In the same way we grow in our faith through obstacles, our marriage also has the opportunity to grow if we choose to embrace the cross of infertility as a couple.

When we are surrounded by friends, especially those who are faithful Catholics with large families, it can be especially challenging. In many Catholic circles, a large family is seen as the norm, and as we struggle with infertility, it can be very hard to see other married couples have their children and continue multiplying their families while we remain barren. As a Catholic, this has a particular bitterness because our society in general does not value a large family the way our Church does. It can be hard to attend Church gatherings where large families are the norm. We can offer up our sadness and remember not to compare ourselves or grow envious of others. Because as spouses we are in this together, we can be a tremendous support to one another in these difficult settings.

Pruned and Shaped

My husband and I have belonged to the parish of St. Timothy ever since we were married. It seems fitting that from Paul's second letter to Timothy we can obtain wisdom for this journey: "Beloved: Bear your share of hardship for the gospel with the strength that comes from God" (2 Tm 1:8b). My husband often says he knows we are stronger because of our experience with infertility. "What doesn't kill you only makes you stronger," he says. I sometimes cringe when he says it, not because I disagree but maybe because of how hard this whole process has been.

In John 15, we read about how God prunes us and how pruning hurts, but it will allow us to bear more and better fruit. As a child I was very blessed to often go on vacation to Disney World, and I remember the beautiful topiaries in the parks. These different figures require a great deal of expert trimming and constant maintenance. Within the pruning process, I came to a point where I felt like I was almost there, almost the shape God wanted me to be, but I had this one branch that needed to be cut that was so stubborn and I just couldn't let it be cut. The fear of what would happen if I did was overwhelming. I knew I was not indifferent to whether or not we got pregnant, and I fought so hard to hang onto that branch. I knew I was fighting it, and all I could do was cry and surrender to God.

I can't say there was a moment where I felt better, but with time, I found the idea of adoption growing more in my heart and I felt the pruning was done for now. All plants need to be constantly pruned, but God also knows when to give us a breather and let us gather our strength. I believe that this pruning has hurt us both intensely, but I see that it has allowed us to bear more fruit, perhaps not the one we wanted but rather the one God wanted. This is the way it happens for most of us, yet we hear more about the dramatic events that occur to others. We are not for the most part converted

Tools to help overcome the difficulties in marriages:

1. Community support—strong friendships are a great help on the journey
2. Counseling and Catholic advice
3. Ministry—serving the Lord
4. Prayer life—maintaining an active prayer life as a couple
5. Continued dialogue—about not only infertility but also other things

like St. Paul but rather gradually pruned and shaped to be more Christlike.

Relax Together

We also need to remember that infertility cannot become our entire lives. We need to continue enjoying each other's company while going on dates and relaxing together. It can be so easy to forget to do this, forget the reasons we are together, but some of the most healing moments can be a simple walk in the park holding hands or a dinner at a favorite restaurant. In the same way that you schedule doctors' appointments and the like, schedule date nights and remember that your relationship is about much more than having children.

Novena Prayer to St. Anne and St. Joachim

Good parents of the Blessed Virgin Mary, grandparents of
   our Savior, Jesus Christ,
When life seems barren, help us to trust in God's mercy.
When we are confused, help us to find the way to God.
When we are lost in the desert, lead us to those whom God
   has called us to love.
When our marriage seems lifeless, show us the eternal youth
   of the Lord.
When we are selfish, teach us to cling only to that which
   lasts.
When we are afraid, help us to trust in God.
When we are ashamed, remind us that we are God's children.
When we sin, lead us to do God's will.
You who know God's will for husband and wife, help us to
   live chastely.
You who know God's will for the family, keep all families
   close to you.
You who suffered without children, intercede for all infertile
   couples.

You who trusted in God's will, help us to respect God's gift of
    fertility.
You who gave birth to the Blessed Mother, inspire couples to
    be co-creators with God.
You who taught the Mother of God, teach us to nurture chil-
    dren in holy instruction.
You whose hearts trusted in God, hear our prayers for . . .
    (*mention your requests here*).
Pray with us for the ministry of Catholic family life.
Pray with us for the ministry of Natural Family Planning.
Pray with us for all who give their time, talent and treasure
    to this good work.
Hail Mary . . . Our Father . . . Glory be . . .
God of our fathers, you gave Saints Anne and Joachim the
    privilege of being the parents of Mary, the mother of
    your incarnate Son. May their prayers help us to attain
    the salvation you have promised to your people.
We ask this through Christ our Lord. Amen.[3]

Further Reading

Guarendi, Ray. *Marriage: Small Steps, Big Rewards*. Cincinnati:
    Servant Books, 2011.

Pastoral Solutions Institute. Home page. Accessed September 18,
    2011. www.exceptionalmarriages.com.

$\mathcal{A}$ Male Perspective on Infertility

So you have failed? You cannot fail. You have not failed; you have gained experience. Forward!

St. Josemaría Escrivá

Men experience infertility differently from women. Alex, Carmen's husband, wrote this chapter so that you can hear a male perspective on infertility and learn from Alex's experience.

Failure and Solutions

When a couple struggles to conceive, a man may see himself as failing to be a provider by not being able to "provide" the desired child or children. I certainly saw myself as a failure in this way. I would often tell my wife I was sorry I could not get her pregnant. I knew rationally this was not my role and that it is ultimately up to God. I took on this burden thinking it was something I was unable to do. As such, I was ascribing too much power to myself and in some way hoping the responsibility would fall on me. "It's not working because of me," is what I would often say. It seemed as if so many couples around us could get pregnant willingly or unwillingly, but not us.

The greatest obstacle for me is the constant, monthly feeling of failing. That big, fat word: failure. Having a clear, known, tangible, attainable, and possible goal each month and not succeeding can be very demoralizing. I quickly become drained and frustrated when I feel like I haven't even come close to conceiving a child. The fact that my wife and I suffer from secondary infertility is particularly challenging. We hadn't had any trouble conceiving before. Why now?

Another frustration for me is the tendency to look for solutions to problems without considering the steps in between. For example, we have a friend who was deemed infertile and told his wife that maybe she should find someone else to have a baby with. This makes sense as a "solution" to the immediate obstacle, but it's not the answer to the real problem. On the other hand, when I didn't know or find any solutions, I blamed myself. Eventually, I realized it is not my fault and that conceiving a child takes three individuals—a husband, a wife, and God. I quickly learned that while my wife and I might be doing our part to be healthy, God has his master plan, which we might never understand or fully realize.

It can also be tempting to be like Hannah's husband, Elkanah, who asked if he was enough for his wife: Her husband Elkanah used to ask her, "Hannah, why are you weeping? Why are you not eating? Why are you so miserable? Am I not better for you than ten sons?" (1 Sm 1:8). I find it helpful to realize that husbands and wives may never understand each other's perspectives perfectly when it comes to infertility, and that's okay.

Test Results and Treatment Options

When we realized after many months of trying to conceive that something wasn't right, my wife was the first to undergo medical screening. Since some hormonal issues were discovered, we concentrated on her. It took close to two years before I had my first semen analysis done. Subsequently, I have had quite a few semen analyses done. Carmen and I were careful to collect the sample using a perforated condom in conformity with Church teaching but found that our chosen method seems to be looked down upon by the lab processing the sample. The andrologist (doctor who analyzes sperm) preferred the sample to be collected in the office and would question our sample's integrity.

Some doctors we visited were also extremely quick to judge us and guide us toward in vitro fertilization (IVF). It seems that with men, doctors automatically move to intrauterine insemination (IUI) or IVF. I remember wishing the doctors would ask if we are in favor of IVF before discussing it as a viable option for us. Recently, a urologist even suggested that my wife was the one who did not want IVF because she did not want to go through all of the hormones and ordeal. When my wife said it was for moral reasons, his said, "Oh, you're very religious." This was simply unnecessary, and doctors should take care to be much more sensitive to people who do not agree with IVF.

Ultimately, the only doctors we found who were willing to honor our beliefs were doctors who believed in Natural Family Planning (NFP) and the teachings of the Catholic Church. All of these doctors happened to be either ob-gyns or doctors of internal medicine. Unfortunately, this was compounded by the fact that there are very few options available for males struggling with infertility. A lot more treatment options exist for women. As such, finding a doctor who specializes in male infertility has been a constant challenge for us. When we did find a doctor for our needs, I was diagnosed with a varicocele (a varicose vein in the scrotum that leads to reduced sperm count and motility). We went to several specialists to see if surgery was necessary or if there were other options. Eventually, we ended up right back with the same doctor with whom I had scheduled surgery previously. In an attempt to avoid confronting reality, I cancelled that scheduled surgery and refused to call the doctors to make follow-up appointments. My wife did not want to push, but I asked her to schedule the surgery because it was too hard for me to do myself. When I finally committed to the surgery, I withheld the news from my parents—I didn't want anyone to know about what I viewed as my "failings".

I recently heard about a couple that experienced infertility and were not satisfied with the natural options, so they opted for IUI and had a child. After a second child came as a surprise, they decided to have a vasectomy, which is a procedure that prevents sperm from being released into a man's semen and is considered a form of permanent birth control. This begs the question of why our selfishness has gotten us to the point where we see children as such a burden. How can the same people who struggled with infertility and were so desperate for a child get to the point of not wanting more?

Frustrations and Consequences

As an architect, if a client comes to me with the desire for a new home, an addition, or a commercial space, I can tell them within a few minutes with 99.9 percent certainty what the zoning and building code requirements are and whether they can build what they would like. While local building regulations are the ultimate authority, I know with a fair amount of certainty if it's possible or just a dream—whether it's a family's dream come true or just an unfulfilled fantasy. Unfortunately, this is not the case with medicine related to male infertility.

I have taken up to twenty-two pills a day for the last several years, and as a result, I often feel impotent, lazy, humble, inefficient, and unhealthy. Not only do these pills serve as a reminder of my infertility, but I have to take some pills with food, some pills in the morning, some at lunchtime, and others at dinner. I am reminded at least three times a day of how infertile I am. Yet, with all of these pills, there are no guarantees that I will improve. This is one of the many frustrations of infertility.

My wife and I are Natural Family Planning instructors, and we try to emphasize the importance of the man's involvement. For years, this was a practice we lived ourselves, but at some point, I stopped being involved with the charting of her monthly cycle. I no longer recorded temperatures or knew what day of the cycle it was. The disappointment of years of unsuccessful attempts was too much, and I avoided it.

In hindsight, I can tell that when the infertility issues weren't about me, I wasn't as emotionally involved, but when the doctors thought that the problem might be with me, things changed.

The Stigma of Male Infertility

On several occasions I have doubted my manliness, or lack thereof, in not being able to conceive a child, and I was often tempted to suppress my feelings surrounding the grief of infertility. I wondered if my masculinity would be called into question if I tell others, especially other men, that I have "abnormal sperm." When all of these doubts cloud my mind, I try to focus on the fact that my measure as a man is not judged by other men—it is judged by God and God alone. God will look inside my heart and see what I have done and, more importantly, how I have done it. I have to remind myself that I am not less manly or masculine due to my infertility. Instead, I adopt the notion that infertility can help me become a better man, better husband, and most importantly, a better child of God. Despite understanding that my masculinity is not defined by my fertility, I struggle to find the courage to talk to fellow husbands and fathers about my pain. I even have close friends who also struggled with infertility, but it was not something we talked about. I had a friend who was told by his father that he was not a real man until he fathered a child.

That is how ingrained in us the idea of virility is. Years later, and even after having children, that statement still hurts him.

Men want to discuss success, not failure, with other men. For men, talking about the situation doesn't help the situation. This philosophy can leave a man feeling isolated. A friend of mine said he would have likely joined an online support group had there been one at the time, partly because of the anonymity it provided. Another man I know felt left out when talking to friends who had kids. He said he "didn't have anybody to talk to." So he chose to emotionally ignore the fact that he and his wife were infertile.

Women may feel comforted by discussing their infertility with friends, hence there is a plethora of Catholic infertility blogs *by* women and really *for* other women. Men, on the other hand, are very private about infertility, especially if there is a male factor causing the infertility. I don't like to talk about myself much in general. I don't want to talk about my infertility with anyone else, much less other men, because I don't want them thinking any less of me. People don't generally like to share their failures, but they love to talk about their many successes or those of their children. I also don't feel comforted by just talking, as I don't feel it's going to improve the situation. Even thinking and writing about it is challenging and humbling for me.

Sexual Frustration

My wife and I have been trying to conceive for over three years now, and we will continue trying. We have always been careful to come together on the day of ovulation, the day after ovulation, two days before and after ovulation, and a slew of other days around Carmen's ovulation, which we know about quite well from our Natural Family Planning training. On many occasions, we abstain for a bit right before we make love to increase my sperm count and potency.

To say that our sexual relationship has taken a bit of a hit is an understatement. In addition to the idea that timing intercourse sometimes makes me feel like I'm being used for my sperm, I no longer feel as hopeful in the idea that our sexual relations will produce a child. I am sexually frustrated, not at the sexual act of intercourse itself or our lovemaking, but at the lack of results from our love. The sexual act is the union of the body and soul in order to help create new life with the help and blessing of God. But I do not feel like a co-creator along with God when I'm not able to help create anything.

Practical tips for men struggling with infertility:

- Pray with your wife and for your wife.
- Pray by yourself.
- Visit the Blessed Sacrament on a regular basis.
- Let go of control of the situation and trust in God.
- Take up a hobby to help keep your mind occupied.
- Exercise and live a healthy lifestyle.

I used to be very frustrated with God about this. I often thought, "I am a good person, a husband, architect, son, and father. Why, then, would God so easily grant me the honor of caring for two of his children and yet deny me the opportunity to be a father to more children?" My tendency is to think, if I am good, or so good, then I should be given whatever I want as if I have earned it. I often feel like Job when he exclaims, "What are my faults and my sins? My misdeeds and my sins make known to me!" (Jb 13:23). However, scripture also reminds me that God has a plan for my family, and I need to trust in that despite what I think I deserve. It's not easy to adopt this mentality, but I do my best to hold on to this hope and faith that God is in control and I am not.

Supporting Your Spouse

How can a woman best support her infertile husband? Pray for him, and be patient and understanding of his differences. For example, it is typical that the wife has read a bazillion articles, books, and online items and is much better informed than the husband. My wife is also a speed-reader, and it was daunting trying to keep up, so I just didn't even try.

A wife can also talk and listen to her husband. If she perhaps cannot provide the support the husband needs, they can find a support group, counselor or friend for him to confide in. Talking does not generally help men in the same manner as it helps women or come as naturally to men, but it nonetheless does help many men.

Letting Go

It was so hard for me to come to terms with my infertility. It was a year after we had our first semen analysis indicating that there may be a problem before I decided to have the surgery to potentially correct my varicocele. Even the doctor told me I took quite a while to decide. As we were leaving the hospital parking lot the day of my surgery, we received a phone call from our adoption agency. We had finished the adoption paperwork and were approved only one week prior to a call informing us we had been matched and our adopted twins were on the way! God literally waited until all was spent, like Abraham and Isaac. He so richly rewarded us after I decided to let go and give all to him. Don't have fear; trust God.

St. Joseph is not someone who is well documented in the Bible, but his holiness is evident. Joseph never had a biological child, yet he is the model for fathers. In fact, in many countries, Father's Day is celebrated on his feast day. I think it is interesting that the saint whose example as a father I should follow is an adoptive or foster father. It shows that being a parent is not about biology alone but also about parenting, which is simply the act of instructing others in the faith and in life. Does a man need to have a biological child to feel like a man? St. Joseph didn't let this distract him from serving God and his family, and I would be doing well if I come close to his example.

Prayer to St. Joseph

St. Joseph, guardian of Jesus and chaste husband of Mary, you passed your life in loving fulfillment of duty. You supported the holy family of Nazareth with the work of your hands. Kindly protect those who trustingly come to you. You know their aspirations, their hardships, their hopes. They look to you because they know you will understand and protect them. You too knew trial, labor and weariness. But amid the worries of material life, your soul was full of deep peace and sang out in true joy through intimacy with God's Son entrusted to you and with Mary, his tender Mother. Assure those you protect that they do not labor alone. Teach them to find Jesus near them and to watch over Him faithfully as you have done. Amen.[1]

Male Supplements

There are many supplements that have been shown to improve semen analysis in different studies. Some of these include the following:[2]

- Transfer Factor Plus Advance, a supplement, available at various websites including www.4life.com and www.4tf.com/products

- Pycnogenol®, 200 mg, resulted in improved sperm quality and function because the natural antioxidant protection was supplemented.

- CoenzymeQ10, 200 mg

- Androvite—multivitamin for men recommended by Marilyn Shannon in *Fertility, Cycles and Nutrition*

- Arginine, 2–4 grams/day

- Taurine, 2–4 grams/day

- Zinc, 50–200 mg/day

- Vitamin E, 400–800 mg/day

- Vitamin C, 1,000–2,000 mg/day

- L-Carnitine, 250 mg[3]

- Captopril

- Folic acid

- Mass cell blockers—antihistamines (tranilast 300 mg or ebastine 10 mg)

- Lycopene, 2,000 mcg 2× a day[4]

$\mathcal{T}$he Loss
of Miscarriage

God remains in you in order to hold you up. You remain
in God in order not to fall.

St. Bede the Venerable

A person's a person no matter how small. This is Horton
the elephant's mantra in the classic children's book by Dr.
Seuss, *Horton Hears a Who*. Though not intended as a pro-life
book, the sentiment repeated throughout this children's book
can also be an anthem for those who suffer the loss of miscarriage. That person was a real person, no matter how early
in the pregnancy the miscarriage occurred. There may be a
tendency by some to minimize miscarriage loss, but the loss
is a death, a very real death of a person, who was a member
of that family.

Miscarriages occur more frequently than we may think.
The statistics vary with as many as 31 percent of pregnancies ending in miscarriage according to a study published in
the *New England Journal of Medicine*, and one in two hundred

resulting in stillbirths. Most experts believe that the number of reported miscarriages is not indicative of the actual number of miscarriages that occur. Many women may miscarry and never know they are pregnant; others may miscarry before implantation and have no way of knowing either.

Miscarriage is defined as the loss of a pregnancy before the twentieth week. After the twentieth week, the loss is classified as a stillbirth. A couple that suffers three or more miscarriages is considered to have recurrent miscarriage.

Many women delay having children because of career decisions, for example, and the incidence of miscarriage increases after age 35. Despite all the advances in medicine, the rate of miscarriage in the United States has remained fairly constant. For many couples, it is surprising to hear how common miscarriage is and that, for the most part, it is nature doing what it is supposed to do.[1] Hearing how common it is can be comforting to the woman who feels alienated because of her experience with miscarriage.

Mourning

The bereavement of a child is unique. It may also seem very unnatural. We all understand that our parents and grandparents will likely die before us, but our children are supposed to outlive us. It is also a loss of the future, the plans we had. The hopes and dreams you had as you planned your future with this child are shattered. Miscarriage is not something you get over or recover from; it changes you, and you will never be the same. It becomes a part of who you are. However, there are certain things you can do that will make it easier to adjust to your new future. During this difficult time, it is helpful to know the five stages of grief:

- Denial—it may take some time to assimilate what has happened. You may be in disbelief for a period.

- Anger—you may get angry with yourself, your spouse, or even God.

- Bargaining or guilt—you may wonder if the situation could have been avoided in some way. You may feel you did something to cause the miscarriage.

- Depression—deep sadness may even lead to clinical depression—you should look for signs of this as discussed in chapter 4.

- Acceptance—you come to a place where you have peace.

I used to think these steps were like a staircase or a ladder that you experience one by one in successive order until you reached the highest one, the best or healthiest one: acceptance. I have since learned that these are actually stages we may move through quickly, slowly, or randomly. One day we may be at acceptance and the next be angry. Grief is a process, not a moment. Healing is attained only by the necessarily slow progression through the stages of grief. It isn't going to be "all better" in a few days or even months. Grief is powerful.

An important thing to keep in mind is that you don't "get past" the loss. Tears will still come, maybe less frequently, but the sadness is still there. Initially, you may be emotionally numb, which can be a coping mechanism. Grieving is also not morbid or a sign of weakness in any way. St. Francis de Sales said, "Have patience with all things, but first of all with yourself." The more we accept that some days will simply be better than others, the easier it will be. Some people may be dismissive of your loss, saying that your grief is excessive for a child you never met (according to them), but this child, no matter how small, was a person and is your child. You are a mother and a father even if you were never able to meet your child.

Grief also has a way of hitting us at unexpected moments, triggered by things we didn't expect. Sometimes we cannot foresee a trigger, but sometimes we know that some activities may be difficult, such as going to a baby shower right after experiencing a loss. You should give yourself time to mourn. It might be wise to politely decline those kinds of invitations until you are ready. Hearing of other babies who have been born or other birth announcements is difficult, especially when the announcements are for babies who were born around the time when your baby was due.

In dealing with grief there are no shortcuts. Going to the hospital to have a postmiscarriage procedure done, for example, can be hard because this is where you thought you would go to have the baby, not lose it. Also, for many women, the procedures themselves are difficult because, in some cases, they are similar to those used in abortions. Eva experienced two miscarriages and had one dilation and curettage (D&C). She shared how hard it was to know that some people voluntarily undergo D&Cs in order to abort children.

Healthcare professionals may think you are crazy for your sadness, but rest assured it is perfectly normal. Jessica shared how one physician refused to perform a dilation and extraction (D&E) on her because she was crying after the loss of her twin boys.[2] The doctor went so far as to order a psychiatric consult for her, as if what she was feeling was out of the norm. Sadly, some doctors become immune to the grief. Fortunately, Jessica was able to find another compassionate doctor to perform the procedure.

We do not have to have a prescribed period of mourning as people used to. It's a process. My mother's brother died in a car accident when he was young, and I have seen pictures of my grandmother in those days, all in black, wearing a picture of her son. To some extent, the prescribed mourning could be viewed as restrictive, but by the same token everyone knew my family was mourning and it was accepted that this was done. Now, people want to "get over" things quickly and simply feel good. They don't want to experience the pain.

A consequence of this, though, is that invalidated grief may lead to depression. It is important to work through the grief. Be patient with yourself, and give yourself time to heal. Over time, the intensity of the grief decreases, and the intervals between episodes increase.

Providentially, as we were writing this book, St. Anthony Messenger published a beautifully written article about miscarriage and infant death entitled "Soul Sisters: A Story of Joy and Sorrow," by Colleen Connell Mitchell.[3] Mitchell describes how she offered her childbearing years to the Lord as a gift and how the loss of her three-month-old son Bryce as he slept, as well as a subsequent miscarriage, challenged her to the core. She describes how she learned to carry her cross of sorrow while living a life full of joy; she says it is the most courageous thing a grieving heart must do. Echoing that sentiment, don't be mad at yourself for feeling joy in your life. Times of joy help heal some of the pain of grief.

A particularly poignant line from this article is "He had designed the family that gave us the best chance to reach our goal, which is to spend eternity in heaven with God." This demonstrates a very Christian perspective on death. It echoes the reality that we are all here only a short time, and our goal is to be in heaven with our Creator. Losing a child can make it very difficult to maintain this perspective.

As we interviewed couples for this book, Susan shared how having three miscarriages changed her views on abortion. She and her husband, Robert, had to trust that God had a plan for them and their children. "We hope to be in heaven with all of our children someday, even those we never saw," Susan said. She and Robert ultimately felt it was their duty to work through organizations like Respect Life to bring about awareness that a pregnancy equals a child.

In my mind, this union with our children in heaven will be like a new dawn. Mourning and morning are homonyms, words that sound the same but have different meanings and spellings, yet the two words are intertwined. When any of us has to travel the valley of mourning, it seems like a long, dark road, but when we continue traveling on the road, however slowly and painfully, eventually we begin to see the sunrise over the darkness and morning comes.

Blame

Anger with God is very common during this time, along with the temptation to blame him. However, blame is never constructive, and it will not help with the healing. You may feel you prayed like you've never prayed before, and he did not answer you. You may feel God has asked you to give back something you were not ready to return. However, there is light at the end of the tunnel, and life will get better as you learn to cope, never losing sight of that special place your child has in your heart. Every child has a soul, and it can be helpful to think about having a special heavenly intercessor for your family now.

It's important to continue communicating with God, even if all you can tell him is how angry you are. Keep that relationship alive. As the C. S. Lewis character in the movie *Shadowlands* said, "I pray because I'm helpless. I pray because the need flows out of me all the time. It doesn't change God. It changes me."[4]

A miscarriage can also seem like a failure, especially of our bodies, and the woman may be very tempted to blame herself. However, it is important to keep in mind that miscarriage is a natural occurrence, and in most cases, there isn't anything she could have done differently to prevent it from happening. Even the word miscarriage seems to imply that something was done incorrectly. The baby was mis-carried. This is an unfortunate nomenclature, but it helps to realize that, in the case of miscarriage, it is usually an issue of compatibility between the sperm and egg, and this happens on a microscopic scale often out of our domain of control.

Infertility and Miscarriage

A miscarriage after many years of infertility may feel cruel in some sense. We may wonder why God allowed this life to begin only to take it away. We may feel it could have been better not to even know we were pregnant. We try so hard sometimes to understand why things happen, and we conjure up all sorts of hypotheses, but in the end, "My thoughts are not your thoughts, nor are your ways my ways—says the Lord" (Is 55:8). We need to trust and let go.

One of the great challenges of miscarriage is the lack of control. For those who experienced infertility, it can be a return to the feelings of helplessness that seemed to have plagued them for so long and that they thought were over with the pregnancy. It is a humbling reminder that life is not within our control. There are expectations many times that we can take a medicine and things will be better, but with miscarriage the doctors simply can't do anything. It is also an opportunity to be reminded of what a miracle life is.

Many women also experience panic attacks following a miscarriage. Counseling may be needed to work through the anxiety attacks. See chapter 4 to see if you have any of the symptoms of depression or anxiety attacks. If so, seek professional help.

My sister-in-law gave my husband and me a beautiful cross-stitch of St. Paul's well-known Corinthians passage on love as a wedding present. From the back, the gift looks like a bunch of haphazardly knotted threads; no words can be read, and none of the images are clear. But when you turn it around, the beauty of the message is clear. Life can be that way. We may not understand why things occur, and our life may simply look like a tangled mess of different colored threads, but on the other side, God is weaving a masterpiece.

Ectopic Pregnancy

It is important to also have the advice of a trusted physician who can adequately inform you about options and treatments. This applies in all cases but is particularly important in the case of an ectopic pregnancy. An ectopic pregnancy is a pregnancy growing outside the uterus. Babies growing outside the uterus do not survive, and if the baby is in the fallopian tube, there is a chance the tube can rupture and cause internal bleeding in the mother, risking her life. Immediate medical attention is extremely important if an ectopic pregnancy is suspected.

In 1970, the Centers for Disease Control and Prevention (CDC) began to record the statistics regarding ectopic pregnancy, reporting 17,800 cases. By 1992, the number of ectopic pregnancies had increased to 108,800.[5]

There are several treatment options for ectopic pregnancies. A salpingostomy is a surgery that removes the embryo through an incision in the wall of the fallopian tube, or a salpingectomy removes either all of the tube or only the part to which the embryo is attached.

For an early-term pregnancy, methotrexate, a medication that can help the body to absorb or pass an ectopic pregnancy, may be administered. The use of methotrexate to treat ectopic pregnancies is still unexamined by the magisterium. Catholic theologians and medical doctors are divided on the issue. *Dignitas Personae* does not take up the morality of using salpingostomy as a treatment for ectopic pregnancy.

However, some doctors may pressure you to take methotrexate or have a linear salpingostomy without determining whether or not the baby was still alive. If the baby has died, there is no moral consideration because there is no taking of life. Also, if a fallopian tube ruptures, both mother and baby are in imminent danger, and if nothing is done both will die. The doctor must act even though only one life can be saved. The rupture is the cause of the baby's death, not any procedure or treatment. The moral predicament arises when life is detected, for example, a heartbeat is found.[6] Because of the lack of clarity on the morality of treatment options for ectopic pregnancies, it may be helpful to seek the help of a Catholic medical ethicist if time allows. A list of Catholic ethicists can be found in the appendix.

Burial and Funeral Rites

One of the most common experiences we heard from couples who experienced the loss of miscarriage and stillbirth was the desire to have a funeral or some sort of ceremony or ritual to remember and offer prayers for the baby and family.[7] No child is too young to receive the Funeral Rite for Infants. Unfortunately, it may be difficult to get a priest to say a Mass for a miscarried child because these are not commonly done, but it is important to stand firm in this desire if it is something you would like because it can bring healing. "Through ecclesiastical funeral rites the Church asks spiritual assistance for the departed, honors their bodies, and at the same time brings the solace of hope to the living."[8] As a Church we proclaim that life begins at conception; we need to back this up with our actions and respect and support families seeking relief from the death of their child, no matter how small. The Church has placed a great deal of importance on burial; as a matter of fact, burying the dead is one of the corporal works of mercy.

Sadly, before twenty weeks most hospitals treat a baby as a lab specimen, and they don't tell families about the option they have to bury the child's remains. Some women even feel lied to about the baby not being a real person since doctors may refer to the baby as a blob or bunch of cells. "The corpses of human embryos and fetuses . . . must be respected just as the remains of other human beings."[9]

It is important to know that an unbaptized, miscarried child can be given a Christian funeral. If the parents intended to baptize their child, the *Code of Canon Law* makes it clear: "As regards funeral rites catechumens are to be considered members of the Christian faithful. The local ordinary can permit children to be given ecclesiastical funeral rites if their parents intended to baptize them but they died before their baptism."[10]

There is a Mass called the Mass of the Innocents or the Mass of the Angels that can be celebrated and that can help bring a spiritual perspective to the sorrow.

Children who have died in utero cannot be baptized, but be reassured that your beloved child is in heaven.

> As regards children who have died without Baptism, the Church can only entrust them to the mercy of God, as she does in her funeral rites for them. Indeed, the great mercy of God who desires that all men should be saved, and Jesus' tenderness toward children which caused him to say: "Let the children come to me, do not hinder them," allow us to hope that there is a way of salvation for children who have died without Baptism. (CCC 1261)

Though it is extremely important for medical professionals and support people to allow the family the chance to make
decisions, the parents may be under duress. Thus, it is important to help the parents make sure that the remains of the
miscarried child be handled with utmost respect. More than
likely, couples will not know anything about how the Church
deals with miscarriage and funeral rites, so we are all encouraged to share this information with couples who miscarry.
Armed with this information, though, the couple must be
allowed to decide how they will proceed and what they feel
will bring most healing to their family.

Catholic parishes and hospitals should provide support to
couples that experience this pain as part of their dedication
to respecting life from the moment of conception. Sometimes
there are no identifiable remains, but when there are, the ritual of the burial and knowing their child is in a specified place
is very important to parents and can bring healing. Burial
policies in the case of a miscarriage vary greatly from state
to state. You may have to work with a pastor or local funeral
home to have your loss recognized and your child's remains
buried. Ask to see if they have reduced rates for miscarriages.
Cemeteries may also have special sections of their grounds
for these children.

In most states, if a baby dies after twenty weeks gestation,
he or she is considered stillborn, and the families must decide
whether to cremate or bury the baby. Stillborn children must
be named and receive a death certificate. Even if your child
died before this requirement, naming the child can be helpful; and even if you don't know the gender, you can choose
gender-neutral names. Name your child and acknowledge
that he or she had a unique identity. By honoring and naming
your child, you maintain a spiritual relationship with a family member who is an intercessor before God's throne, a part
of the communion of saints. Call your child by name in your
prayers and look forward to reuniting in heaven.

If you experienced a miscarriage in the past and were
unable to celebrate a Mass, offer one on the anniversary of

the death of your child. You may also consider offering a community Mass for miscarried and stillborn children. This can benefit other families as well as be a source of comfort for each other (see the end of the chapter for further resources).

Comfort in God's Word

Prayer can also bring about healing. You may take comfort in God's word. Psalm 139 can be helpful as a meditation during this time. Jeremiah 1:5 says, "Before I formed you in the womb I knew you, before you were born I dedicated you, a prophet to the nations I appointed you." Scripture has powerful pleas of sorrow that can be very comforting.

> My soul is deprived of peace,
>> I have forgotten what happiness is;
> I tell myself my future is lost,
>> all that I hoped for from the Lord.
> The thought of my homeless poverty is wormwood and gall;
> Remembering it over and over leaves my soul downcast
>> within me.
> But I will call this to mind,
>> as my reason to have hope:
> The favors of the Lord are not exhausted,
>> his mercies are not spent;
> They are renewed each morning,
>> so great is his faithfulness.
> My portion is the Lord, says my soul;
>> therefore will I hope in him.
> Good is the Lord to one who waits for him,
>> to the soul that seeks him;
> It is good to hope in silence for the saving help of the Lord.

Lamentations 3:17–26

Knowing you now have a saint in heaven can bring you comfort. Knowing there is a special intercessor for your family can be a healing perspective. Eva recommends asking God not why this happened but what he wants you to learn from this experience. Having been through a loss makes us more compassionate toward others. The reminders of the frailty of life can also impact how we view other areas of our existence.

"We do not want you to be unaware, brothers, about those who have fallen asleep, so that you may not grieve like the rest, who have no hope" (1 Thes 4:13). In our grief, however, we should remember the Christian message of hope that St. Paul extols. We know there is hope: our children are in heaven, and we will hopefully meet them one day soon. "But do not ignore this one fact, beloved, that with the Lord one day is like a thousand years and a thousand years like one day" (2 Pt 3:8).

Mary Knows Our Pain

Our Lady of Sorrows is a title we often associate with Mary because of the immense suffering she endured with the death of her son. We have also probably seen many images of Mary crying. When I went to the movie theater to see *The Passion of the Christ*, I was most moved by Mary. I could not control my sobs as I saw her pain. Mary knows what it is like to lose a child. Asking for her intercession can prove helpful. The "Seven Sorrows of Mary," a popular Catholic devotion, might help.

One of the scripture texts I return to frequently for meditation is Luke 2:19: "And Mary kept all these things, reflecting on them in her heart." How did she do it? Simeon told her that a sword would pierce her heart, and yet she treasured all of the life she had with Jesus. Even knowing the little that she did could not have prepared her for what they did to her Son, but her steadfast faith did. We can learn so much from Mary in the face of sorrow and death. Mary, pray for us.

Seeking Support

Many people do not know how to offer comfort to couples that have experienced a miscarriage. I know of a couple who, after hearing of friends who miscarried, said they didn't want to see them because they did not know what they would say to them. Sometimes simply saying, "I don't know what to say," and meaning it is comforting because it shows an effort to empathize. Tell your loved one you are praying for them, as this affirms their loss and shows you care.

People may also be dismissive and say things like "you can try again," thereby not giving value to the life that was lost and that you would like so badly to recover. Children are unique and irreplaceable. The fact that someone may be able to have other children does not lessen the grief of losing this one.

"It was God's will. It was part of God's plan." People say clichés like this to try to comfort us. Though they may be true, they may not help the grieving family. We all want to believe that everything happens for a reason, even if we cannot understand the reason. We want to believe that pain will be justified with some future reward, that God will make everything better.

We also cannot judge how much grief anyone should have. For example, saying that an early miscarriage should be grieved less than a stillbirth is not helpful but instead hurtful. Every situation is different, and we should not fall into the temptation of comparisons. An early miscarriage does not afford the parents the opportunity to see and hold their child, which some feel helps in the bereavement process.

It is important for you, as grieving families, to be honest with those around you so they can help you. Putting on a brave front for family and friends is not helpful. In order for loved ones to effectively help, they need to know what is going on and how you are feeling. Let them know what they can and cannot help you with. For example, sometimes people may want to make decisions for you, to spare you the difficulty of making funeral arrangements, for example, but grieving cannot begin until the loss is real and making choices helps cement the reality of the loss.

Trying Again

Seeking a pregnancy right after a loss may be difficult on our bodies, and this is why most doctors recommend waiting several months before trying to conceive again. Use this time to heal. Some people may think a new pregnancy will help heal the hurt, that it will make you forget the hurt. But grief and our emotions affect our bodies, and stress impacts us in many different ways. The decision to try again is very personal and private, but it is important to keep these things in mind. Also remember that a new pregnancy does not make the sorrow go away. People are not replaceable. If you are pregnant soon after a miscarriage, it is important to take care of yourself, physically and emotionally. You should rest, eat well, and pray.

Blessed John Paul II said not to be afraid, and too often I find myself afraid, afraid that I will not like what God is doing with my life because it is not what I asked for. Fear paralyzes us and can keep us from trying again. We can have fear that future pregnancies will also end the same way. "In life, you can choose to have fear or faith," I heard someone say once, and I thought that was simple and yet so profound. It's our choice to let go of the fear and have faith that, whatever the outcome, it's in God's hands.

A subsequent pregnancy can also heighten any concerns. You may worry about every little pain or breathe a sigh of relief when you go to the bathroom and do not see blood, or you may have fear when going to an ultrasound. Recurrent miscarriage can make this problem seem especially insurmountable. Yet studies have shown that women who miscarry three times and become pregnant again carry to term, up to 70 percent of the time.

There are many reasons a miscarriage can occur, and few doctors specialize in this area. Even miscarriage clinics are rare. Miscarriage clinics strongly encourage testing for chromosomal abnormalities called karyotyping. This information can help couples understand what options and treatments they have available. Half of all miscarriages are due to a chromosomal abnormality, most of which occur within the first trimester. Understanding what caused a miscarriage can also help with the emotional healing.

Your Spouse

Women and men will experience a miscarriage differently. One of you may want to talk about the baby, while the other may prefer to withdraw. Be open and honest with each other as you deal with your feelings. It's important to remember that husband and wife do not need to feel the same things. Grieving is very individual, and everyone's experience of grief is different.

Patron Saints to Invoke against Miscarriages

- Catherine of Siena
- Catherine of Sweden
- Our Lady of Guadalupe, Patroness of the Unborn

This may affect your marriage. You may grow resentful of each other or even blame one another. Jessica shared how miscarriage can affect your sexual intimacy as a couple because of the temptation to view that intimacy as the place where the whole dark road of grief and loss started. Counseling may be beneficial in this case. Ignoring these problems and feelings is not constructive. Joining a support group with other couples may help.

It is important to be supportive of each other; for Jessica, having her husband in the room with her prior to a procedure was helpful. Karla shared, "When you miscarry, you have to talk and pray a lot with your spouse. We had to be on the same page. Talking about it brought us closer together. Also important is relying on other couples who have gone through it, people who understand."

Ways to Remember

Remembering your child in a tangible way is another way to promote healing. The options for these are endless, and you should choose what most resonates with you. Here are some ideas, some of which may or may not be applicable to your situation:

- Plant a tree or flowering plant. This can be symbolic of your child's eternal life in heaven.

- Invest in something physical you can touch—a memory box or blanket, for example. Creating a memory box can also be helpful to store any sympathy cards from friends, ultrasound photos, pictures, and so on.

- Ask for the intercession of your child's patron saint. You can also buy a medal of the saint to wear as a reminder.

- Ask the hospital staff to make handprints or footprints.

- Swaddle the baby or take photos with him or her.

- Keep a journal. Writing your feelings out can be therapeutic. You may choose to write to your child as well—poems, letters, and so forth.

- Create a basket filled with baby items to donate to the local Respect Life center in honor of your child in heaven. This is a beautiful way to give back to the community while treasuring your child's memory.

- Have a Christmas ornament made for your child.

Support a family who has experienced a loss in this way:
- Most importantly, treat the situation as a real death.

- Create a spiritual bouquet—a bouquet with prayer intentions.

- Call or e-mail. Contact the person, letting him or her know you are there.

- Send a sympathy card, perhaps a card offering a Mass.

- Make a meal or send a gift card to a restaurant so they do not have to worry about cooking.

- Make a care package with items that can bring comfort—devotional books, chocolates, treats, and so on.

- Offer to make calls for them to let others know what has happened.

- If they have other children, offer to take the children out for the day or a few hours. For example, offer to take them to school or to an extracurricular activity.

- Help arrange a funeral Mass and burial—call funeral homes and cemeteries for the family. Help them gather the information they need to make the most informed decision possible.

- Help with mundane tasks like paying bills, walking the dog, cleaning dishes, and so forth.

- Offer to listen, if they want to talk.

- Remember and offer a Mass during All Souls' Day.

- Organize a prayer chain of friends who will intercede for the family during their difficult time.

- Remember the anniversary of the baby's death and when the baby was supposed to be born.

- Protect them from hearing other people's horror stories.

- Be patient. Grief takes time.

Prayers

Eternal Father,
Hear the cry of parents who mourn the loss of their child.
Still the anguish of their hearts with a peace beyond all understanding
Through the intercession of the Blessed Virgin Mary.
Mother of all tenderness and our Mother,
Strengthen our faith in you.
Give them Consolation to believe
that their child is now living in the Lord.
We ask this through Christ our Lord, who conquered sin and death,

and who lives and reigns with you, in the unity of the Holy Spirit,
One God, for ever and ever, Amen.[11]

Blessing of a Couple after a Miscarriage

For those who trust in God,
in the pain and sorrow there is consolation,
in the face of despair there is hope,
in the midst of death there is life.
. . . As we mourn the death of your child
we place ourselves in the hands of God
and ask for strength, for healing and for love.[12]

Miscarriage Prayer

My Lord, the baby is dead! Why, my Lord—dare I ask why? It will not hear the whisper of the wind or see the beauty of its parents' face—it will not see the beauty of Your creation or the flame of a sunrise. Why, my Lord?

"Why, My child—do you ask 'why'? Well, I will tell you why.

"You see, the child lives. Instead of the wind he hears the sound of angels singing before My throne. Instead of the beauty that passes he sees everlasting Beauty—he sees My face. He was created and lived a short time so the image of his parents imprinted on his face may stand before Me as their personal intercessor. He knows secrets of heaven unknown to men on earth. He laughs with a special joy that only the innocent possess. My ways are not the ways of man. I create for My Kingdom and each creature fills a place in that Kingdom that could not be filled by another. He was created for My joy and his parents' merits. He has never seen pain or sin. He has never felt hunger or pain. I breathed a soul into a seed, made it grow and called it forth."

I am humbled before you, my Lord, for questioning Your wisdom, goodness, and love. I speak as a fool—forgive me. I acknowledge Your sovereign rights over life and death. I thank You for the life that began for so short a time to enjoy so long an Eternity.[13]

Terms You Should Know

androgen levels. Blood tests to measure male hormone levels.

antiphosphotidylserine, PAI-1 levels, MTHFR, prothrombin II mutation, and Factor V leiden. Blood-clotting tests that may indicate an increased risk of forming blood clots in the small blood vessels of the placenta, which may interfere with continuation of the pregnancy.

blighted ovum. A fertilized egg that died.

dilation and curettage (D&C). Procedure involving the dilation of the cervix and the removal of the child. Most common treatment for first-trimester miscarriage.

dilation and extraction (D&E). Second-trimester procedure, similar to D&C.

endometrial biopsy. A minor surgical procedure to sample the uterine lining (endometrium) approximately twelve days after the urine LH surge indicates impending ovulation; this may show whether the uterine lining has appropriately developed to support a pregnancy.

fasting insulin levels. A blood test to determine whether you have insulin resistance, which may increase the risk of miscarriage.

leukocyte antibody detection and embryotoxic factor. Blood tests to determine whether your immune system is attacking the pregnancy.

ovarian reserve screening. A blood test done at a certain point in your cycle to see if your eggs are too old to function reliably.

perinatal death. The death of a baby from the twentieth week of gestation through the twenty-eighth day after birth.

saline hysterosonogram. An ultrasound test in which a small amount of salt water is injected into the uterine cavity during a scan; this may show uterine scar tissue, polyps, or other anomalies that may interfere with growth of the pregnancy.

stillbirth. Pregnancy loss after twenty weeks' gestation at which point babies may sustain life outside the womb for a brief time.

TSH and prolactin levels. Blood tests for hormone levels that indicate whether your thyroid and pituitary glands are functioning properly.[14]

Online Resources

Elizabeth Ministry:
www.elizabethministry.com/files/Burial_Shows_Reverence_For_Miscarried_Baby.pdf; www.elizabethministry.com/Miscarriage_Child_Loss.html

Faces of Loss, Faces of Hope:
http://facesofloss.com
A website where people can post their stories

Heaven's Gain:
www.heavensgain.com
You can acquire a small casket from Heaven's Gain.

I Am the Face:
www.iamtheface.org
Creates awareness of October 15 National Pregnancy and Infant Loss Awareness Day.

La Belle Dame:
www.labelledame.com/miscarriage-infant-loss.html
Infant and miscarriage loss jewelry

Mayo Clinic:
www.mayoclinic.com/health/miscarriage/DS01105

Medline Plus:
www.nlm.nih.gov/medlineplus/ency/article/000895.htm

Memorials on Eden Hill:
https://secure.marianweb.net/memorialsonedenhill.org/sothi/create.php

Memorial tile for the Shrine of the Holy Innocents at the National Shrine of the Divine Mercy. All children memorialized at the shrine and their families will be remembered daily in the Rosary for Life, in the Holy Mass, and during the Hour of Great Mercy at the National Shrine of the Divine Mercy and in special Masses on December 12 (Feast of Our Lady of Guadalupe), December 28 (Feast of the Holy Innocents), and on the third Saturday in July.

Miscarriage Support:

www.miscarriagesupport.com

Details and stories from other parents who have lost their young preborn children

Morning Light Ministry:

www.morninglightministry.org

A Catholic ministry for bereaved parents; can request a prayer card for your baby

My Forever Child:

www.myforeverchild.com/store/Default.asp

Keepsakes that may help with healing

Now I Lay Me Down to Sleep:

www.nowilaymedowntosleep.org/locate_photographer

Offers free professional remembrance photography for families experiencing a loss as a step in the healing process

Share: Pregnancy and Infant Loss Support:

www.nationalshare.org; www.nationalshare.org/support resources.html

Has local support groups throughout the country as well as resources and training for support providers

The Shrine of the Holy Innocents:

www.innocents.com/shrine.asp

You can have your baby's name inscribed in the "Book of Life" at the Shrine of the Holy Innocents in New York City. A candle is lit in loving memory. On the first Monday of every month, a Mass is celebrated in honor of these children. The shrine will e-mail you a "Certificate of Life" with your baby's name included.

Unborn Jesus:

www.unbornjesus.com

You can have your baby's name inscribed in the Holy Innocents Virtual Mausoleum.[15]

Miscarriage Clinics:

St. Mary's Hospital Save the Baby Unit, London:
www.savethebabyunit.org
The world's largest clinic dedicated to miscarriage prevention.

University of Chicago Recurrent Pregnancy Loss Program:
www.uchospitals.edu/specialties/obgyn/pregnancy-loss

Further Reading

Cohen, Janice, D.S.W., and Gail Owens. *Molly's Rosebush*. Morton Grove, IL: A. Whitman, 1994.

(A children's book on miscarriage.)

Cohen, Jon. *Coming to Term: Uncovering the Truth about Miscarriage*. Boston: Houghton Mifflin, 2005.

(Offers a comprehensive look at the scientific research done on miscarriage along with stories of many couples that experienced miscarriage.)

Kellett, Mary. "Peter's Story: Discovering Hope and Love After an Adverse Prenatal Diagnosis." 2007. www.catechism.org/pro life/programs/rlp/Kellett.pdf.

Otremba, Maureen, and Jim Otremba. "Miscarriage." Accessed September 20, 2011. http://foryourmarriage.org/ everymarriage/overcoming-obstacles/miscarriage.

Schermerhorn, Caroline. "Miscarriage: Moving from Grief toward Healing." *St. Anthony Messenger*, January 2005. www .americancatholic.org/messenger/Jan2005/feature3.asp.

Sodergren, Andrew J. "Hope for Healing: Miscarriage and the Dignity of the Human Body." January 12, 2005. www .christendom-awake.org/pages/may/hopeforhealing.htm.

Wicker, Kate. "Short Lives That Are Long Remembered: Coping with the Loss of Miscarriage." *Faith and Family*, Spring 2011.

Pastoral Resources

Archdiocese of Boston. "Worship and Spiritual Life: Pastoral Notes on the Celebration of Liturgical Rites for Deceased Infants and Stillborn or Miscarried Infants." Accessed September 20, 2011. www.bostoncatholic.org/Offices-And-Services/Office Detail.aspx?id = 12540&pid = 464.

    Resource for priests and ministers helping bereaved families.

"Blessing of Parents After a Miscarriage." In *Book of Blessings*, by International Commission on English in the Liturgy, A Joint Commission of Catholic Bishops' Conferences. Collegeville, MN: Liturgical Press, 1989. www.catholicculture.org/culture/liturgicalyear/prayers/view.cfm?id = 711.

    Parishes and dioceses can hold a day of reflection and an infant memorial Mass for families who have lost a child to miscarriage, stillbirth, or neonatal death.

Articles on the Ethics of Ectopic Pregnancy Treatments

Theologians' views on methotrexate:

- William E. May; Rev. Benedict Ashley, O.P.; and Rev. Albert Moraczewski, O.P., are in favor of its morality.

- Charles Cavagnaro, Thomas W. Hilgers, and Bernard Nathanson reject its use as a form of treatment in these situations.

Catholics United for the Faith. "Ectopic for Discussion: A Catholic Approach to Tubal Pregnancies." Last updated September 26, 2007. www.cuf.org/faithfacts/details_view.asp?ffID = 57.

Howard, Joseph C., Jr. "Personhood: The Moral Management of Ectopic Pregnancies." American Bioethics Advisory Commission. 1999. www.all.org/abac/jch003.htm.

Kaczor, Christopher. "The Ethics of Ectopic Pregnancy: A Critical Reconsideration of Salpingostomy and Methotrexate." *Linacre Quarterly* 76, no. 3 (August 2009): 265–82.

Moraczewski, Albert S. "Managing Tubal Pregnancies: Part I." *Ethics and Medics* 21, no. 6 (June 1996): 3–4.

Chapter 11

*H*ow Family and Friends Can Help

We are not called by God to do extraordinary things but to do ordinary things with extraordinary love.

Jean Vanier

While my husband and I were waiting month after month for God to bless us with a child, I used to say I wouldn't wish infertility on my worst enemy. I probably should have specified that I wouldn't wish it on my best friends, either.

While sharing the experience of infertility with Carmen and Alex, I became acutely aware of the need for greater sensitivity and compassion for those struggling with infertility. Infertility can be a lonely and isolating place, particularly if you don't personally know anyone who has experienced it or is experiencing it (which admittedly is rare nowadays). But it is possible to have supportive family and friends who may or may not have firsthand experience with fertility issues but are still empathetic and compassionate.

> The community of believers is called to shed light upon and support the suffering of those who are unable to fulfill their legitimate aspiration to motherhood and fatherhood. Spouses who find themselves in this sad situation are called to find in it an opportunity for sharing in a particular way in the Lord's Cross, the source of spiritual fruitfulness. (*DV* 8)

This chapter is dedicated to helping family and friends—and by extension, the Church—be increasingly sensitive to those struggling with infertility and treatments.

What Not to Say

Well-meaning people often don't know what to say to couples living with infertility. People have the best intentions, but we all know where those can lead! Here are some of my "favorite" things *not* to say to infertile couples:

- "Just relax—you're too stressed."

  People don't become less stressed by being told to be less stressed. Most times, infertility is caused by an underlying medical issue, not stress. Plus, that implies no one who is stressed conceives, which simply isn't true.

- "Give up; leave it in God's hands."

  The implication here is that one is not detached enough, which is like saying it is somehow the couple's fault because they are not abandoned to God's will. We never know the interior of someone's heart and cannot assume they are not allowing God to be in control.

- "I completely understand how you feel."

  Whether or not you have experienced infertility, everyone's feelings and experiences are different. With empathy, perhaps we have an inkling of what they're going through but not exactly. "I can see how you might feel that way" is a better alternative.

- "Just adopt; there are plenty of kids who need homes."

Yes, adoption is a good option, but coming to terms with this and grieving about never having biological children takes time. Also, not everyone is able to adopt, due to financial reasons or age, for example. As a friend or relative, you may present adoption as an alternative to consider but not as a solution to infertility. If God is calling a couple to adopt, he will guide them to it in time.

- "I was able to conceive by drinking pineapple juice." (or other similar old wives' tales)

We are bombarded by quick fixes to fertility issues. It's already hard not to be tempted to try every solution under the sun. Saying what worked for you merely adds stress to the couple trying to conceive.

- "I got pregnant when I wasn't even trying."

This kind of comment can be hurtful and implies that not trying is the solution. With the gift of Natural Family Planning, it is often hard for couples not to try given how we know our most fertile times each month.

- "Why are you trying some unknown Catholic treatment when so-and-so got pregnant easily using in vitro fertilization (IVF)?"

It is hard enough to face many secular doctors who question our desire to remain true to Church teachings; we don't need our family and friends questioning us, too. Instead, ask questions about the treatments, not out of mere curiosity, but to be more informed on the myriad options available to Catholics. You never know when you can pass along the information to someone else.

- Saying nothing.

Ignoring the problem or denying it exists isn't being a good friend. Simply because the couple isn't talking about it doesn't mean you don't need to address it. People should always be given the option to talk about their infertility journey; if they choose not to, then respect that and remind them you are there for them. You may follow up with them at a future point when they feel more ready to talk about it. But by all means, don't pretend it doesn't exist; this is like ignoring the elephant in the room. This only serves to minimize it. And if you don't know what to say to your infertile friend at any given point, simply express, "I don't know what to say right now but count on my prayers." At least it's understood that you care and you're trying.

So what should we say or do to help our loved ones carry the cross of infertility? Believe it or not, some of the right words come straight from God's Word.

On Holy Ground

While tending to his father-in-law's flock one day, Moses saw a strange sight: a bush that was on fire but was not consumed. Moses heard God calling to him from the bush, and as Moses answered and approached, God said to him, "Remove the sandals from your feet, for the place where you stand is holy ground" (Ex 3:2–5).

Similarly, though it may be challenging to bear this cross, the flames of infertility will not consume our infertile family or friends. It may be intimidating for us to approach them because seeing our loved ones going through refining fire can be tough, but we must remove our sandals and listen to what they have to say. To remove our sandals is to take ourselves out of the equation, leave behind our assumptions and pre-judgments about infertility, and ask the Holy Spirit to help us be present to our loved ones. Removing our own sandals also enables us to place ourselves in another's shoes in order to enable us to be more empathetic.

Each person's experience with infertility is sacred, holy ground because that is where God is sanctifying them. That said, we must tread lightly and merely walk with them, sandals cast aside. If we have experienced infertility in the past and we are supporting a friend who is currently experiencing it, we cannot expect for them to feel the exact same things we felt. Some feelings may be similar, and we can draw from this to relate to their experience, but others may be new or particular to their individual situation. God works through different people in varied ways, and we should be careful not to interfere with God's work in them.

Moses feared the burning bush, but the message he received from the Lord through this bush changed his life forever. Similarly, we may fear approaching our loved ones and may not know what to say or do, but it is in this holy space, this holy ground, that God resides. Offer to pray for your relatives or friends, ask them if there is a specific intention you can pray for. Print out or e-mail them some of the prayers listed in this book to encourage them. Remember that prayer doesn't necessarily change God, but prayer can change your loved ones.

Being a Good Samaritan

Imagine walking along a well-traveled path and finding a man, beat up, by the side of the road. What will you do? Walk on by, because you're afraid or too busy, or stop and do what you can to help him out? In Jesus' parable of the Good Samaritan, the Samaritan traveler is "moved with compassion" for the injured man and, after bandaging his wounds, "took him to an inn and cared for him." The Samaritan treated the stranger with "mercy," and Jesus calls us to "go and do likewise" (Lk 10:25–37).

In his apostolic letter *Salvifici Doloris*, Blessed John Paul II explains that the parable of the Good Samaritan teaches us about the relationship we have with each other as we suffer: "We are not allowed to 'pass by on the other side' indifferently; we must 'stop' beside him. Everyone who stops beside the suffering of another person, whatever form it may take, is a Good Samaritan. This stopping does not mean curiosity but availability."[1]

Christ is showing us through this parable the importance of suffering with someone. As the pope explains, this sensitivity of heart (empathy) must be cultivated. This may not come naturally to some of us, but through effort, it can be achieved.

The Good Samaritan does not just sympathize and have compassion toward the injured man; note that what moves him is not pity but mercy and compassion. Pity is a dangerous emotion that can be inadvertently conveyed to our infertile loved ones through patronizing looks or words. We're not called to feel sorry for them; we're called to empathetically love and support them as the Good Samaritan did in giving of himself.

"Here we touch upon one of the key-points of all Christian anthropology. Man cannot 'fully find himself except through a sincere gift of himself.' A Good Samaritan *is the person capable of* exactly *such a gift of self.*"[2]

Suffering, then, is "present in order *to unleash love in the human person,* that unselfish gift of one's 'I' on behalf of other people, especially those who suffer."[3] Love is what compels us to help those who are suffering. In the case of our friends going through infertility, we can write them little cards or give them meaningful religious gifts (prayer cards, Mass intentions, crucifixes, inexpensive statues or jewelry, etc.) to remind them of God's love. Take them out for coffee (or better yet, ice cream or cupcakes!) and then pay a visit to the Blessed Sacrament together to pray before our Lord. These little acts of kindness will not remove the pain but maybe help them not focus on it, even for a little while.

Helping to Bear the Cross

Knowing I had friends willing to walk with me through infertility helped me to remain sane and focused on God. I know how much my friends wished things were different, and I'm sure we wish our family and friends wouldn't have to suffer through this either. We desperately want them to leave behind the cross of infertility, but our faith in them and in God helps them to bear their cross with grace.

While Jesus was carrying his cross to Golgotha, Simon of Cyrene was ordered to help him carry the cross. Some have postulated that Simon was chosen because he may have shown sympathy with Jesus, though it is generally thought he had no choice. The movie *The Passion of the Christ* portrays Simon of Cyrene as a Jewish man who was forced by the Romans to carry the cross, and though at first he was unwilling, he eventually showed compassion for Jesus as they journeyed together to Calvary.

We all have suffering and we all carry different crosses, but our suffering can unite us. Even if you have never experienced infertility, at some point, each of us has felt the need to be cared for or felt the emptiness of loss. Empathy does not require us to have identical journeys, just the ability to put ourselves in the place of the suffering individual and realize how difficult their journey is. Once we have taken that step to truly try to understand their circumstance, we are moved by God's love and compassion.

How can we help them bear their cross? Although you can't physically remove their cross or completely carry it for them, maybe offering up to God our own stresses, ailments, or illnesses on their behalf for their pain of infertility can help unite our suffering. "People who suffer become similar to one another through the analogy of their situation, the trial of their destiny, or through their need for understanding and care, and perhaps above all through the persistent question of the meaning of suffering."[4]

You can also offer to do online research on their condition and seek possible treatments in line with Church teaching. If we, as supporters, are informed, we are better able to serve as a support system. Offer to drive them to appointments, or if they have other children, offer to take care of them while they go to their appointments. If their sense of despair is particularly acute, lovingly suggest that they meet with a Catholic therapist, priest, religious, or spiritual director in order to work through the negative emotions and find hope in Christ. The most important thing is to ask how you can help. You never know what would be most helpful to them and their situation.

Standing at the Foot of the Cross

I have always been struck by the contrast in the number of friends Jesus had and the number of friends who actually stood by him in his darkest hour. The only ones at the cross were his mother, Mary the wife of Clopas, Mary Magdalene, and John, who is referred to as the "beloved disciple." By being present at the foot of the cross, Jesus' friends demonstrated great compassion, which is a word used today without much thought. By definition, *com-passion* is to be *with* someone in their time of *passion*—to suffer with them. If we share in our loved ones' suffering, we demonstrate our commitment to them and our love for their family.

But what about the disciples who didn't show up at the foot of the cross? Where were his friends when Jesus needed them most? I have often wondered what went through his disciples' minds to make them decide not to accompany him. Maybe something to the effect of "this is too hard to bear—I can't stand to watch"; "this doesn't concern me—I shouldn't get involved"; or "I'll pray for him, but there's nothing I can do."

Standing at the foot of the cross requires fidelity and courage. Everyone else turned away from Jesus on the cross. We may have friends who would rather avoid us than deal with the suffering. I have heard of people who purposely avoided someone experiencing infertility because they didn't know what to say. These friends can be challenged and most especially prayed for so they can grow in their ability to empathize.

Who knows if I would have made the same decision to not stand by Jesus at the foot of the cross. I would like to think I would have been there for my friend as John was: "When Jesus saw his mother and the disciple there whom he loved, he said to his mother, 'Woman, behold, your son.' Then he said to the disciple, 'Behold, your mother.' And from that hour the disciple took her into his home" (Jn 19:26–27).

Speak and Act with Love

For those who know and love infertile couples, don't feel that you have to say much; just being present and listening is enough because there really isn't much to say. What could Mary and John possibly say to Jesus while at the foot of the cross? Don't undervalue the power of empathy. Sometimes, there just isn't much we can say, and nothing we can do can remove this cross. But just being there, enabling our family members or friends to vent and feel understood, can be a huge help.

There are so many emotions associated with infertility: so many hopes and so much anxiety, so many doubts and uncertainties. Caregivers and people helping those experiencing this cross should be sensitive to this and consider this before speaking. It's not about walking on eggshells around them but rather about measuring our words carefully in the light of compassion.

When we don't think before speaking and don't word things carefully, we may come off as insensitive, which in turn denotes a certain indifference to the situation. Because infertility is a different type of suffering than a physical pain or perhaps the death of a loved one, people can unintentionally minimize the extent of the suffering by way of an insensitive or dismissive comment.

Saying things like "You should really move on" or "The moment I let go, I got pregnant," for example, can be hurtful and insensitive. Because I've been there and experienced hurtful comments firsthand, I make extra efforts to phrase things in a sensitive way when speaking to couples going through infertility. This requires thinking before speaking, which is extremely important for supporting infertile couples.

Despite my best efforts to be as sensitive as possible, I may inadvertently phrase things in an insensitive way. The key is to apologize and make a better effort next time. Just because the comment or question was not well phrased or well received does not mean you should never inquire again.

Special care should be given when announcing pregnancies to infertile friends or family members. Sometimes an in-person announcement of a pregnancy may not be received in the best way. As discussed in chapter 6, other peoples' pregnancies are indeed a source of joy but also often a reminder of what is not transpiring and is so sought after for the infertile couple. Though it may seem impersonal or contrary to what one might expect, e-mail might be the best option to announce a pregnancy rather than a verbal announcement. E-mail affords recipients of the good news the opportunity to react in their own way and, once they are done processing and praying about it, respond in a more appropriate, joyful way than what might have been their initial reaction in person. Others may have other preferences, though, so if you anticipate a pregnancy announcement soon and you want to be sensitive to your infertile friends, perhaps ask them if they have a preference as to how to be told.

Similarly, when extending invitations to baptisms or baby showers, a mailed invitation or e-mail would also be most appropriate. It can be difficult to continuously attend showers and baptisms (as is apt to happen in the twenty- to forty-something age range), and if a couple chooses not to attend a particular baby shower or baptism, please know it is not personal. We don't know what particularly difficult moment along the infertility journey they may be experiencing at that moment.

Life changes in many respects when families have children, and it is important to not leave out the infertile couple, particularly when everyone around them seems to have children but them. Though families with children tend to have events that center around the children (birthday parties, etc.), be sure to take some time every so often to get a babysitter and go out to dinner or play board games with your friends experiencing infertility.

Also, be careful what you discuss in the presence of infertile couples. It's a given that people in this age bracket often talk about pregnancy, children, and parenting. But talking about this all night at a dinner party in the presence of someone struggling with infertility could be difficult and uncomfortable. Also, be wary of complaining about the challenges of parenting around couples trying to conceive. As Laura Flaherty, founder of Hannah's Heart Catholic Infertility Support Group, says, "It would be kind of like complaining about how tired you are after a night of dancing to a friend in a wheelchair."[5]

The contemporary Christian group Jars of Clay has a song called "O Come and Mourn with Me Awhile," and the lyrics are appropriate in that they contain the message that infertile couples would like their supporters to know. Please come and mourn with us—mourn our infertility awhile, just sit with us and listen, let us feel what we feel. "O come together," the song says, and it's a reminder that suffering together can actually bring people closer together. When we speak, we should speak with love, as with Jesus' "seven words of love." And as the song says, "victory remains with love," so in loving us during this time, we will be victorious over the sorrow.

A Word on Guilt

I remember distinctly that, when I found out I was pregnant with my second son (my first biological son), I had a tough time telling the news to some friends with whom we had been journeying through infertility. I just didn't know how to tell them, and I felt a tremendous amount of guilt.

Even though I was happy, to some extent, my guilt stemmed from wishing I was the one who was hearing the news and not telling it. I wished I could trade places with my friends because of how much I loved them and wanted to see them pregnant as well. Nevertheless, feeling guilty is not a fruitful emotion, and it does not change the circumstances.

I remember reading years later that feeling guilty is not healthy because it somehow assumes that the one who feels guilty is in a better position or is somehow superior. I am certainly no better than anyone else, nor do I think my situation is better than anyone else's. God knows what he does and in the time that he does it.

If you have journeyed through infertility, you may have a tremendous amount of joy in finding out you are pregnant, but there is still a need for sensitivity when sharing the news with others who are struggling to conceive. That said, you should not feel guilty; the fact that you are pregnant doesn't make your experience better than your friends', just different.

Challenging Others to Follow Church Teaching

So what if our family or friends are Catholics who are leaning toward pursuing in vitro fertilization, insemination, or other illicit Assisted Reproductive Technology (ART)? For starters, we can't assume they know what the Church teaches on the subject. If people don't actively seek out Church teaching, they may not know what the Church says on the subject of ART, much less why. Direct them to this book or to the United States Conference of Catholic Bishops (USCCB) literature on what the Church teaches on ART. Many of the Church's documents on the subject are mentioned throughout this book. They may not intentionally want to be going against Church teaching: perhaps they just do not know what Church teaching is; many do not even know that Catholic treatments even exist. It is our responsibility as Catholics to gently direct them to Catholic resources and treatments. Part of being supportive is to also make sure people know there are alternatives that won't compromise their morals.

I know the temptation is always there to not say anything because it seems like it's none of our business. Who enjoys confrontation or putting ourselves out there? I, for one, have a physical reaction to challenging people: I actually tremble in fear! But the Lord reminds us, "Do not be afraid." I don't enjoy doing it, but I know it is a necessary part of

"The church community cannot take away your tears, but can show you how to make them holy. They can offer you comfort and ways to help mourn your pain. . . . Your doctors may be your guides to needed physical healing, but your faith community will be the guide for spiritual healing and direction."[6]

friendship to occasionally challenge my friends along their faith journey, just as I would want to be challenged if I were going astray.

I'm sure Nathan debated and struggled with having to challenge his friend King David (2 Sm 12:1–13) after David's wrongdoing in taking another's wife and having her husband killed. Nathan could have defended or justified his friend's wrongdoing in the same way we could justify our friends' use of ART to achieve pregnancy. Instead, though, Nathan was a true friend to David and was willing to take a risk in order to redirect his friend to the paths of the Lord. David, in turn, could have responded with bitterness or resentment, but he knew it was his friend's courage and love for him that compelled Nathan to challenge him. It was this love that produced repentance and a return to the Lord.

If you are a priest or a counselor, explain why the Church teaches what it does, that it is born out of love for its children and not out of a desire to control. Unfortunately, I have heard of several cases of priests telling parishioners who come to them for advice in the area of infertility that they should do whatever their consciences tell them to do. The issue with this is we're assuming that everyone's consciences are both formed *and* informed. Indeed, we can't force anyone to make a moral decision, but we can ensure they have all the information presented to them in order to make a proper decision.

Friends in Stormy Weather

As our strength is tried, knowing we have others who support us, on whose strength we can rely, makes all the difference. After all, we're called to "bear one another's burdens" (Gal 6:2). When Carmen first started coming to terms with the fact that getting pregnant was not going to be so easy, I gave her a card that expressed the feeling we have as friends watching our loved ones suffer:

> I wish I had a big yellow umbrella to keep all the rain out of your life.

I would hold it over your head and the drops would splash,
    splash
and you would never even feel them.
But I don't have a big yellow umbrella . . .
    so I'll walk through the rain with you.

As much as we wish we could, we can't stop the rain from falling or even pretend to understand God's plans for each person, but what we can do is walk together. God does not intend for anyone to walk alone, and it is extremely important that those undergoing infertility can find a support system willing to get soaked with them as they weather infertility. Sirach 6:14 says, "A faithful friend is a sturdy shelter; he who finds one finds a treasure." This is the kind of friend we should strive to be.

As Holley Gerth says in her blog, we're more vulnerable when we're alone. "It seems tornados often form quickly on wide-open plains. The same can happen with our hearts and minds." The way to combat this vulnerability of loneliness is to "surround ourselves with people who will encourage and support us. Hint: the best way to find those people is to be one." If infertile couples aren't given the proper space to vent and be encouraged, they may experience residual bitterness that lasts far beyond the infertility experience, as evidenced by a middle-aged neighbor of a friend of ours who was visibly upset by our friend announcing her third pregnancy. The woman had one grown son but had always wanted more children. Infertile couples need not only space to process their pain but also a support network with which to share it.

This also brings to light the pain of secondary infertility as this woman experienced. Sometimes, people without children may inadvertently see those saddened by secondary infertility as selfish or greedy because they already have a child or multiple children yet desire more. We need to be careful not to be judgmental or make comparisons in thinking our own personal situations are worse. Please remember that people experiencing secondary infertility already know firsthand the blessing of children and often feel called by God to continue to grow their families. It can also be hard or surprising when conceiving may not have been a challenge at the outset to then have to face challenges conceiving future children. We should all have greater compassion and understanding for those experiencing secondary infertility.

Probably the most important thing we can do for our friends is to pray for them, not just for them to have a child, but also that God may give them the grace to continue to bear their cross. Pray for them to find redemptive purpose in this challenging journey.

As Christians, we are called to be both fair-weather and foul-weather friends. "He who is a friend is always a friend, and a brother is born for the time of stress" (Prv 17:17), therefore, we become like family to one another during trying times. Though it's not really about us, walking with someone along the road of infertility can be a time of growth for us, too. We can see the ways in which God is working through the lives of our friends with infertility and can learn from their experiences.

The most loving and fruitful things we can do for our friends who carry the cross of infertility is walk with them and pray for them.

Laura Flaherty, founder of Hannah's Heart Catholic Infertility Support Group in Jacksonville, Florida, shared this poignant description of what it feels like to be infertile:

> I want all the mothers who have never struggled with infertility to imagine for a minute that you are unable to have children. Your house is silent; there are no toys or little clothes scattered about. There are no sloppy kisses or "I love yous" whispered from tiny voices. If you're a stay-at-home mom, you are out of a job. You may have a career outside the house, maybe even a career that you love, but it's not the one you want and every day you go to work crying out to God that surely He has called you

to something more than this. You have absolutely no idea
what the future holds. If you're anything like me, you have
always been comforted by the fact that, with enough hard
work and dedication, you can accomplish anything . . . a
strong and happy marriage, a rich spiritual life, a college
degree, home ownership, a promotion at work, etc. However, no matter what you do or how hard you try, you may
never succeed at getting pregnant. And, unlike many trials
in life, where the passage of time is a great healer, even
that is less certain with infertility. With most other trials,
you can say to yourself, "In six months I will have more
resolution and will feel better than I do today." However,
infertility is nothing like that. In six months or a year or
even two or three or more years, you may still have no
resolution and you may feel worse than you do today.[8]

Prayer to Blessed John Paul II for a Friend

Dear John Paul II, servant of God, who are already in
heaven, this is a novena for your intercession that
_____ becomes pregnant and delivers a healthy baby who
will glorify and praise God.

For people, certain things are impossible to attain and sometimes people are unable to understand God's will, but we
deeply believe in your intercession, John Paul II. You always
defended children, especially the unborn ones and you loved
them above all. Please look at _____ who is asking for
children. Look at the tears in her eyes, begging to become a
mother.

St. Anne, you gave birth at a late age to our Queen of heaven
and earth, the Most Holy Mary. That is what God wanted.
With God nothing is impossible. We believe that God, Creator
of heaven and earth will look kindly upon _____ and
give her the blessing, through Mary, the Virgin Mother of God

and John Paul II, of becoming a mother of her biological and adopted children whom she will love and thank God for.

Dear John Paul II, please help our prayers to be answered and that _____'s womb will be filled with the beating heart of a tiny baby. We already give you thanks and sincerely believe in your intercession.

Dear John Paul II, your beloved mother also asked God for you to be born. Please remember our prayers. Amen.[7]

How Parishes and Dioceses Can Support Infertile Couples:

- In Prayers of the Faithful intentions, include mothers and fathers who long to bear children but are struggling with infertility, especially on Mother's Day and Father's Day.

- Incorporate infertility awareness within marriage preparation.

- Start an infertility support group.

- Celebrate Masses annually to specifically pray for couples experiencing infertility and the loss of miscarriage.

- Increase diocesan-wide awareness of Natural Family Planning and the Catholic alternatives to Assisted Reproductive Technologies, possibly through widely publicized speaking engagements with Catholic doctors.

- Create care packages that include prayer cards, a St. Gerard booklet and handkerchief, Mass intentions, and a brochure on Catholic treatment options for parishioners suffering from infertility. The Elizabeth Ministry and St. Gerard Store (links found in chapter 7) sell wonderful low-cost items to include in these packages that can help support couples.

"Couples who face incurable infertility and those who choose adoption need the same pastoral compassion and support, just as [do] those who seek reconciliation for turning to immoral treatments during the emotional rollercoaster.

"Right now many couples seek help from treatment centers who dangle statistics and 'experts' who offer hope. The more the topic of infertility is ignored, the more couples will choose the option they feel has the most to offer them. We need to be the place they look to for hope."[9]

Tips for infertile couples:

- Be patient with your family and friends. Though they may sometimes say hurtful things, they do have your best intentions at heart.

- Prepare a well-rehearsed response to insensitive comments. For example, "We want children but are having trouble. We are seeing a specialist and ask for your prayers. We prefer not to talk about it."

- Many people simply don't know what the Church teaches on infertility, nor that there are Catholic treatment options. Though it can be hard not to get defensive, showing them the resources you have learned may help them to be not only more informed but possibly more sensitive.

- If your family and friends challenge you in love, listen to the heart of the message more than the delivery of the message. They may just not know how to phrase it appropriately, but the message could be one of love and concern.

- Pray for those who are supporting you, that God may help them to be empathetic and loving toward all those experiencing infertility.

$\mathcal{O}$pting
to Adopt

In love he destined us for adoption to himself through
Jesus Christ, in accord with the favor of his will.

Ephesians 1:4–5

I know a little boy who could have been the victim of abortion. He was born in a small village in Vietnam named Viet Tri in August 2006. In 2000, Vietnam was the country with the highest number of abortions in the world—there were 1.4 million abortions in Vietnam in 2005. To give you an idea of the culture of death and encouraged abortions in Vietnam, in 2007, there were more abortions than births in Ho Chi Minh City (previously Saigon).

Nevertheless, according to the little information provided, this child's birth mother was a young woman about twenty years old. She left him at a medical clinic when he was about three days old so that others could take care of him and give him a better life than what she could offer him. No one knows for certain what her motivations were, but she chose life for her son.

This child is now our son, Emmanuel Cuong, and we never could have imagined for ourselves when we began our infertility journey that such a tremendous blessing was prepared for us by God.

A Call to Adoption

As Christians, we are all called to adoption in some way or form. "Religion that is pure and undefiled before God and the Father is this: to care for orphans and widows in their affliction" (Jas 1:27). Each of us may be called in different ways to do this. For some, this call may involve welcoming an orphan into our homes through fostering or adoption; for others, this could mean a spiritual adoption of a child (or widow) who needs our prayers, encouragement, or monetary support.

According to the catechism, spouses who suffer from infertility after exhausting legitimate (and acceptable) medical procedures should unite themselves with the Lord's Cross and "give expression to their generosity by adopting abandoned children or performing demanding services for others" (*CCC* 2379).

Some people discern that they do not want to live a child-free life and try to adopt, while others may discern that they are called to more ministry or service in the Church or other areas of need. A life without children can still lead to a good, fruitful life in service of the Lord.

However, adoption is a wonderful, loving option that should be at the very least considered, discerned, and prayed about. The Lord will guide you and your spouse as to whether or not adoption is for your family. In adoption, you may experience parenthood not how you first may have imagined it but certainly fully. Through adoption, couples can cooperate with God in raising children for him, which ultimately should be our goal. We should not want children for our sake but rather for their sake, as their own people with equal dignity to us.

Jesus' description of the Last Judgment in Matthew 25 also mentions that "I was a stranger and you welcomed me. . . . Whatever you did for one of these least brothers of mine, you did for me." To welcome a child into our homes is to serve Jesus in the least of our brothers. This does not, however, mean that a child we adopted is worth any less than we are or than a biological child is worth—it just means that "whoever receives one child such as this in my name, receives me; and whoever receives me, receives not me but the one who sent me" (Mk 9:37).

Though adoption may seem to be a modern phenomenon, there are numerous instances of adoption in scripture. Moses is one such example.

> It was his birthmother, acting for fear of his life and trusting God's intervention, who placed him in the basket in the river. And it was Pharaoh's sister, after discovering the abandoned child afloat on the water, who brought him to her brother where he was raised as Pharaoh's own son. It was in this adoptive environment that Moses learned the leadership skills necessary to lead the Israelites from slavery in Egypt to freedom.[1]

Esther was also adopted, by her cousin, Hadassah. "The girl was beautifully formed and lovely to behold. On the death of her father and mother, Mordecai had taken her as his own daughter" (Est 2:7). She grew to be the queen of Persia, and God used her to bring deliverance to the Jewish people.

Finally, Jesus himself had St. Joseph as his adoptive father. Although not much is said about Joseph in scripture, we know he initially had doubts, but he trusted in Mary and in God (I'm sure it helped that an angel appeared to him to set his mind at ease) and raised Jesus as his own son. He never fathered a biological child, but he rearranged his life unselfishly to help Mary and held such an important role as an adoptive father.

Perhaps it can help to think of our own adoption journeys after infertility in much the same way. Maybe we come to adoption through a process of elimination—it's the only choice left. However, we do not know what God is planning with our lives. In thinking about Mary and Joseph, we are reminded of how even God did not come in the way he was expected to and how Mary's plans were really rather scary. Yet God is always at work crafting his plans with love.

For us, adoption is probably not anything we would ever have seriously considered for our family were it not for our unexplained infertility. It certainly involved a lot of trust to just go where God guided, and some days, I just felt like I was going kicking and screaming. But God is our loving Father who knows what we need more than we do, and just like with Mary and Joseph, he provided all that we needed.

In addition to being called to adoption, the Bible and catechism also remind us that we, too, are adopted. "For those who are led by the Spirit of God are children of God. For you did not receive a spirit of slavery to fall back into fear, but you received a spirit of adoption, through which we cry, 'Abba, Father!' The Spirit itself bears witness with our spirit that we are children of God" (Rom 8:14–17). What a beautiful image to know that even though God is not our biological father, we are able to call him Daddy because he has adopted us as his own.

The very first verses of the catechism also state that we are adopted children of God. "When the fullness of time had come, God sent his Son as Redeemer and Savior. In his Son and through him, he invites men to become, in the Holy Spirit, his adopted children and thus heirs of his blessed life" (*CCC* 1). We inherit a blessed life in him just by the mere fact of being God's adopted children—how humbling this is. And yet, it is this blessed life that we have inherited without merit that impels us to ensure that our children—no matter how they come into our families—share in this life in Christ. "We can invoke God as 'Father' because the Son of God made man has revealed him to us. In this Son, through Baptism, we are incorporated and adopted as sons of God" (*CCC* 2798).

Baptism is when we are officially welcomed into our Church family. When Emmanuel came home from Vietnam in April 2007, we threw him a big party with all of our family and friends. Baptism, in turn, is a welcome home party that God throws for us as he celebrates our adoption into the Church as his beloved child.

Kinds of Adoption

As of the 2000 Census, there were 1.5 million children under age 18 in America who joined their family through adoption, which accounts for 2 percent of all children in the United States. There are more than five million people today in the United States who were adopted, and a total of about one hundred thousand children are adopted domestically and internationally each year by US parents.[2]

There are three major categories of adoption: adoption through foster care, domestic adoption, and international adoption.

Foster Care

Foster care is the term used for a system in which a minor who has been made a ward (ie, when his or her care is given to the state) is placed in the private home of a state-certified caregiver referred to as a foster parent. The state, via the family court and child protection agency, makes all legal decisions while the foster parent is responsible for the day-to-day care of said minor. The foster parents are paid by the state for their services.

The Health and Human Services report from the Adoption and Foster Care Analysis and Reporting System (AFCARS) reported that 55,684 children were adopted from foster care in 2009, an increase over previous years.[3] Nevertheless, there is still a need to find families for the more than 114,000 children in the US foster care system that are eligible for adoption.[4]

The cost of adopting from foster care tends to be relatively low, up to $2,500.[5] Foster care is intended to be a short-term situation until a permanent placement can be made. There are three options for permanent placement: (1) reunification with the biological parent(s), when it is deemed in the child's best interest (ie, parents stop using drugs, show proof of having attended detox and remain clean, etc.); (2) adoption; (3) permanent transfer of guardianship—tends to happen with older children, as in the case of the movie *The Blind Side*, in which the Tuohy family took over the guardianship of Michael Oher, a high school–aged ward of the state (later turned NFL football player) who was essentially homeless due to his biological mother's drug use.

In an ideal world, all children would remain with their biological parents, but sometimes this isn't possible, due to death of the parents, illness, lack of resources, addictions, improper care of the child, and so on. My favorite line from the movie *The Blind Side* is when a friend of the family tells Leigh Anne Tuohy, the adoptive mother, "I think what you are doing is so great, to open up your home to him. Honey, you are changing that boy's life," to which Tuohy responds, "No, he's changing mine."

Though I have not been a foster parent, I can certainly relate to the misconception that taking in a child in need is purely altruistic. Several people have told us how lucky Emmanuel is to be in our family. Sure, it's answering a call from God to care for an orphan, but in the end, we're the lucky ones who have the humbling privilege to raise one of God's own, and in so doing, we are changed for the better.

"In order to come to the aid of the many infertile couples who want to have children, adoption should be encouraged, promoted and facilitated by appropriate legislation so that the many children who lack parents may receive a home that will contribute to their human development."[6]

Domestic Adoption

The National Council for Adoption (NCFA) reports that domestic adoption has increased in recent years. In 2007, 133,737 domestic adoptions were reported, an increase of 2.6 percent over the reported 130,269 domestic adoptions in 2002.[7] The number of domestic infant adoptions varies from year to year, but it has been on the decline since 1992.

There were only 18,078 domestic infant adoptions in 2007 (the most recent year for which the study was able to obtain statistics), compared to 22,291 in 2002. This 18.9 percent decrease indicates that proper counseling and education to encourage adoption as an option needs to continue to be given to women facing unplanned pregnancies.[8]

Most people in the United States who adopt domestically adopt infants, many of them newborns that they are able to pick up from the hospital. I have a few friends who were present for their baby's birth. A huge advantage of domestic adoption is that the baby can be with you practically from day one. Whether you adopt an infant or an older child, you are likely to receive more extensive history and background information about a child who lives in the United States than one adopted internationally.

The typical wait time for domestic adoption is about one to two years, though a recent poll conducted by *Adoptive Families* magazine found that 76 percent of domestic adoptions took one year or less.[9] In most US newborn adoptions, adoptive parents are selected by the birth parents of the child, and, in at least half of the cases, the birth parents and adoptive parents have met. Birth parents usually have forty-eight hours after the child is born to sign off on their legal parental rights, while some states require birth mothers to wait thirty to forty-five days after giving birth before relinquishing parental rights. Once the adoption is finalized, the adoptive family is recognized as the child's family by law.

In domestic adoption, families may choose to work with a public agency, a licensed private agency, an attorney (independent adoption), or an adoption facilitator or unlicensed agency (if allowed by laws in your state). Public and licensed private agencies are required to meet state standards and have more oversight to ensure quality services. Unlicensed agencies and facilitators often do not have the same state oversight, so there may be more financial, emotional, and legal risk for adoptive and birth families using unlicensed services. Many public and private adoption agencies offer free orientation

sessions that will allow you to gain an overview of their available services prior to making any commitment to work with
them.[10] Costs of domestic adoption vary greatly depending
upon the type of agency used but can range anywhere from
five thousand up to forty thousand dollars or more.[11] Some
domestic adoption agencies are nonprofits with sliding scales
based on income.

There are various levels of openness in domestic adoption.
Open, or fully disclosed, adoptions allow adoptive parents,
and often the adopted child, to interact directly with birth
parents even after the adoption is finalized. Family members interact in ways that feel most comfortable to them and
may include letters, e-mails, telephone calls, or visits. The
frequency of contact is negotiated and can range from every
few years to several times a month or more. In semi-open or
mediated adoptions, contact between birth and adoptive families is made through a mediator (e.g., an agency caseworker
or attorney) rather than directly, and very minimal identifying information is exchanged. In confidential or closed adoptions, no contact takes place and no identifying information
is exchanged.[12] Closed adoptions are seldom done anymore;
the norm is more often open or semi-open adoptions.

International Adoption

The modern era of international adoption began after
the Korean War, when Korean and Amerasian orphans were
placed with families living in the United States. Since then,
Americans have adopted many thousands of children from
Africa, Asia, Eastern Europe, and Latin America.

There has been a significant decline in intercountry adoption in recent years. There were 11,059 immigrant orphan
adoptions reported in 2010. In 2007, the year we adopted
Emmanuel, he was one of 19,608 children adopted abroad.[13]
The figures from 2010 are even more surprising when noting
the overall five-year decline of 51.7 percent since 2004, when
22,900 intercountry adoptions were reported. The dramatic

decline in the number of intercountry adoptions can be attributed to a variety of factors, many outside the control of US adoption officials and advocates. Adoption has slowed or shut down in many countries, for reasons that vary across countries; "the most common reasons include concerns about corruption, the slower processing of adoption cases, an increased focus on domestic adoption programs within sending countries, and stricter regulations on which children are eligible for adoption."[14]

Another factor contributing to decreased international adoptions is the enactment of the Hague Convention on the Protection of Children and Co-operation in Respect of Inter-Country Adoption, which entered into force in the United States in April 2008. The Hague Convention is "an international agreement to establish safeguards to ensure that intercountry adoptions take place in the best interests of the child."[15] The Hague Convention basically started to discourage so-called baby buying (illicit buying and selling of babies to profit from adoptions) and helps ensure that adoptions are safe and ethical. The Hague Adoption Convention applies to adoptions between the United States and the other countries that are signatories.

Typical wait times for international adoption have traditionally been one to two years, though nowadays, due to the Hague Convention, wait times may be longer since investigations are more thorough. In some countries, families are required to travel to meet the child beforehand, or have to visit with the child first, depending on the rules of the country. I have often been asked how we came to choose Emmanuel to adopt, and I explain that our private agency and the orphanage worked together to assign children to adoptive families—adoptive parents don't go to an orphanage to choose their child.

Costs for international adoptions also vary greatly, ranging from seven to thirty thousand dollars (but generally more toward the upper end of that spectrum).[16] There must be an intercountry adoption agreement between the United States and the adopting country in order to be able to adopt from that country; one can't just adopt from any country. Countries open and close adoptions depending on politics and ethics. Adoptions to Vietnam, for example, have opened and closed throughout the years. Vietnam opened shortly before we adopted from there and closed shortly thereafter—they were only open for about a year and a half, and we were able to adopt in that short window. South Korean adoptions will soon close, and Guatemala closed right before we adopted. Perhaps these countries will open again in the future—or other countries will open. It's all hard to predict.[17]

Coming to Terms with Our Adoption Fears

Carmen says that, from a young age, she always felt called to adoption, and before marrying Alex, they discussed this being a part of their family. When it came time to actually adopt, however, the process proved to be much harder than anticipated. "Doubts filled my mind: What if this was not what God wanted? What if we were forcing the issue of children and were not humbly accepting God's will and plans for our family?" she questioned. She shares that one of her favorite Bible passages is "Perfect love casts out fear" (1 Jn 4:18:). "Despite my knowing this passage and what it meant, fear of making the wrong decision plagued me. Sharing the fears with God and knowing that he will help us overcome them has been helpful because the fears do not completely subside, they may change, but they come back all too often."

What Carmen describes is all too common, and there is no shame in feeling or sharing these fears and doubts. Adoption is an uncharted territory for most people, and the unknown always come with, well, the unknown.

Many couples begin the adoption process without first dealing with or coming to peace with their infertility. Perhaps it's the seeming finality thereof that is difficult to accept, but to some degree, couples need to grieve and accept the loss of a biological child, despite knowing that God can make all things possible. Entering the adoption process can seem like we're giving up on hope of biological children, and there may be a sense of anger or resentment at having reached this point. There may also be a sense of hope that, perhaps not in nine months after beginning the process but eventually, you could become parents—that is pretty amazing in its own right. God can help us work through these mixed emotions of anger and hope and prepare us for the road ahead.

There is an often-perpetrated myth that, once one starts the adoption process and starts focusing on that or "relaxing" to some extent, a couple will become pregnant. (Many of you have probably been told this firsthand.) Ironically, even though we did become pregnant in the process of adoption, I still don't believe this myth because it can be damaging and could lead couples to pursue adoption in order to get pregnant (perhaps subconsciously) and not because it is a decision they feel called to regardless. Starting the adoption process cannot be viewed as another form of treatment for infertility.

After adopting their second of three children from Colombia, our friends Elise and Matthew said a family member inappropriately asked them why they didn't have their own kids. Apparently, they had a family member tell them to "stop adopting and just have your own. Do I need to show you how it's done?" You hear a lot of strange things, but what he said took the cake.

Another favorite comment people tell infertile couples is "Well, if you don't get pregnant you can just adopt." This seems so simple to those not struggling with infertility, and this statement dramatically minimizes adoption and the calling to adopt.

Commenting on a blog post on infertility, Sarah said, "Adopted children are not the consolation prize of the infertile. Couples adopt a child because they are open to life and God leads them to it."[18] Becoming a family through adoption is in no way superior or inferior to biology—it's just different, in the same way that God created us men and women, different but of equal dignity. An adopted child is not a substitute for a biological child but a person who needs love and caring; he or she is an individual loved by God in the same way as any other person.

Unfortunately, others may feel that adoption *is* a substitute for a pregnancy, hence the use of terms like paper pregnancy to describe adoption (due to all the paperwork that must be completed) and the parallels of wait and expectation, though the waiting is different from that of pregnancy. Sometimes, friends who desire to be supportive may bring up your adoption process during a conversation involving pregnancy or children, and this may be frustrating, because it is being perceived as the same. It's okay to feel that, though you are anticipating having a child through adoption, you find that your desire to have a child be the fruit of your love for one another is not diminished. A Catholic infertility blogger at *This Cross I Embrace* posted that "we do a great disservice to adoption when we automatically connect it to infertility, and don't honor it for the beautiful and amazing blessing it is on its own. Logically, our human minds will always connect the two. But in our words and actions, they should remain two separate and distinct entities."[19]

Because they are two separate entities, they should be discerned as such. As I explained in chapter 5 on discernment, I want to underscore the importance of being informed in order to make a proper decision about adoption. For starters, deciding to adopt was not an impulsive decision we made on a whim. We researched and prayed a lot. We did not arbitrarily choose a country from which to adopt, for example. We read up on each country's adoption programs (the ones that were available for adoption at the time), general information about the health of children from each country, and so forth. Then we used this research (intellect) and joined them to our feelings (affectivity) in order to arrive at a decision that God blessed.

Discernment needs to include both husband and wife communicating where the Spirit is guiding. For example, Alex had a stronger calling toward domestic adoption than did Carmen. Carmen had done research in school and always had a place in her heart for Chinese girls and their plight. Once it came time for them to potentially adopt, they discussed it many times. For them as for us, there was not one instantaneous moment of clarity that we were called to adopt, it was more of a gradual leading and guiding of the Spirit. Adoption is done by choice and out of love. Many Christians refer to it as having a heart for adoption.

Adoption is the path that God chose for our family, but it is not necessarily everyone's calling. Some people would love to adopt but may not qualify to do so for any number of reasons including factors such as age, past criminal record, or medical history.

> Adoption may not be an option for some people. It may be impeded by the lack of a baby to adopt or other factors, or a couple may rightly judge that their negative feelings toward adopting would make it too risky for a prospective adopted child, and so rule it out. Still, every married couple can exercise their capacity for parenting by helping other parents in some way or by doing other things analogous to parenting, such as helping to care for the handicapped or elderly people who cannot care for themselves or need help in doing so.[20]

The blogger at *This Cross I Embrace* continues,

> Some childless couples will feel the call to adopt. Others may not get that call, and may instead feel called to childless living. Still others may receive the call to adopt many years from now. And some may have a surprise pregnancy in their future, in God's time. Each plan is paved out by God, and each plan is specific to those two people.

> This is what God wants to do for each individual couple . . . who suffers with infertility/childlessness. He wants us to deepen our faith, grow in His love, and become His hands on earth. Our focus as humans should not be on a pregnancy or an adoption as the "result" at the end of the

infertile couple's suffering, but rather, on life everlasting.
Should a couple adopt children or conceive after years of
infertility, all glory and praise be to He who gives life—but
these are blessings only, NOT the Resurrection of the cross
of childlessness. Our Resurrection will come in heaven,
not on this earth.[21]

Adoption requires surrender. It means trusting that, if
you're called to adopt, God has a special child, or children,
out there for you and that he will bring you together as a
family. There are so many stories we may have heard about
how an adopted child came into a particular home, and just
as God knows how to deal with each of us in the most appropriate way he will see to it that the process yields the desired
outcome.

Preparing for Adoption: Carmen's Story

As a child, I loved watching The Sound of Music. I remember they would put it on TV every year around Easter time—
my favorite holiday—and I would ask for permission to stay
up to watch it. I remember the Mother Superior telling Maria
(Julie Andrews) that when God closes a door somewhere he
opens a window.

I've often felt that God guides our lives through the opening and closing of doors and windows, opportunities that present themselves and those that do not as well. At the point in
which I felt the possibility of biological children was a closed
door, adoption became the window that brought fresh air and
perspective to our struggle. For us, it was also just one window
that was opened.

We had decided that in the same way we sought Catholic
treatment for infertility, we wanted to pursue an adoption
through a faith-based agency. In our area, Catholic Charities
no longer does adoptions, so we looked to Christian agencies
within our state. It was shocking to discover that we were dis-
criminated against because of our Catholic beliefs and flat-out
told by various agencies that they would not place children

in our home because we are Catholic. It was very sobering to feel that once again our options were being limited by our religious beliefs, but instead of viewing it negatively we chose to see it as God helping us narrow down an overwhelming number of options and literally leaving us with just one agency—an agency whose mission is to save children from being aborted, which was recommended by friends. From the very beginning, it was clear that this was where we needed to be.

The Adoption Process

The adoption process can be very intimidating and emotional. One thinks that having children will be an intimate personal decision, but the path of adoption is much more public. The degree of scrutiny can feel intrusive and unsettling at times. Backgrounds will be checked, homes inspected, references contacted, intimate and personal questions asked, and fingerprints completed—it's not for the faint of heart. With steps such as the home study (where a social worker visits your home to inspect it and interview you) and birth-mother letters and sometimes even websites, adoption can feel like we need to market ourselves, like we have to convince someone that we are good enough to be parents. But the preparation is important, and when you're willing to jump through all these hoops for the sake of parenting a child, God can work through this preparation to help confirm our call to adoption. The thing to remember is that, ultimately, the entire adoption process is up to God, just like in a pregnancy.

The counseling and the process of preparing for adoption can be painful but is necessary to deal with the emotions and prejudices buried in our subconscious that we do not even realize we have. Our adoption agency did not require any adoption preparation other than mailing us a spiral-bound book on international adoption, which we read and was helpful to some extent but did not go far enough. We signed up for a local adoption parenting class, read books and took a few online adoptive parenting classes that were also supportive, but we still felt unprepared for what lay ahead. In fact, sometimes reading too many things without the appropriate guidance or direction from a social worker, for example, can be detrimental because you can inevitably read more about what can end up going wrong in adoption (which is not all that common) and less about everything that can go right.

The agency from which Alex and Carmen chose to adopt required reading several books and writing reports on them as part of the preparation for adoption. Some may feel this is an unnecessary step and may resent it because they feel biological parents have no such requirements, but "the requirements were very much a part of my healing and my cross," said Carmen. "It was hard (and I mean hard) to read the books, hard to write a birthmother letter, hard to write a profile marketing ourselves to potential birth mothers. I would work on these requirements piecemeal because the emotions would take over after a bit and I would have to take time to process. But therein was the beauty: I was forced to, by virtue of the hoops we had to jump through, process and continue processing. It's amazing how we think we're done with something, that we've overcome an emotion, and then something will set us off."

Although in-depth preparation as required by an agency can be challenging, I commend their agency for doing what they do and encourage you to find an agency that also has stringent adoption-preparation requirements. I really wish we were more mentally and emotionally prepared for adoption. You can also pretty safely deduce that, if an agency is going to such great lengths to prepare you for adoption, they are likely going to equal lengths to prepare birth parents, too, which is another huge benefit. If your agency doesn't have many requirements to prepare you for adoption, sign up for a class locally or online and ask your social worker or agency plenty of questions.

Birth Parents

I must confess that one of the many reasons international adoption was appealing at the time we adopted our son is because of the anonymity it afforded of no contact with his birth family. With time, though, I have come to realize that this anonymity is a double-edged sword. We have absolutely no medical history for our son (though he's healthy as a horse) and barely any information about his birth mother. Now that he's beginning to ask questions about his adoption (and will likely continue to do so through the years), we really wish we had more information to share with him about his family background. Given the nature of international adoption, however, we will likely never know. We pray for his birth mother with such gratitude for her supreme gift and offer her up to the Lord's care because we know that she is known and loved by him.

As I mentioned previously, Carmen and Alex had to prepare for their domestic adoption by reading books, several of which were about birth mothers. Carmen shared how deeply this impacted her:

> I had never put too much thought into birth mothers and what they go through, but the more I learned, the more I realized how incredibly selfless placing a child for adoption is. As a teenager teaching the Confraternity of Christian Doctrine (CCD), I remember teaching my students that the definition of the word sacrifice was "a special gift of love." Birth mothers make a remarkable sacrifice for their children, and adopted children need to be made aware of how much they were loved by their birth mothers. They make this sacrifice for the greater good.

This also reminds us of Mary. The Church teaches us that Mary's fiat included some understanding of the suffering she would endure, and yet she said yes. These families suffer, these mothers suffer, but they say yes to a better life for their children. We need to pray that more women and families are willing to be so selfless and loving.

Adoption Risks

Adoption is full of joy and tremendous blessings, but like pregnancy and childbirth, it is not without risk. The window of time that birth parents have to relinquish their parental rights varies by state. Domestic adoptions are sometimes not final until the last minute or even for many months after placement. Needless to say, if birth parents change their minds about proceeding with adoption, it can be heartbreaking for adoptive parents who have been planning for the child's arrival into their homes. The loss and grieving involved is said to be similar to that of miscarriage. If you have suffered the pain of adoption loss, here are some tips to help you get through it:

- Allow yourself to grieve the loss.

- Failed adoption is a significant loss and it is important to recognize it as such. Allow yourself time and space to mourn.

- Be patient with your spouse, who may grieve in his/her own way.

- Each of us processes loss in different ways. Be patient with one another and keep the lines of communication open. It may help to pray and spend more time together.

- Accept the loss and ask God for the strength to continue and the guidance to know how to proceed.
  After an adoption loss, it may be hard to know how to proceed—whether to pursue another adoption and, if so, how soon. Pray for God's guidance in this area.

- Allow your family and friends to help and support you.
  They may not know exactly what to say, but they want to support you. Let them know how they can best help you, either by cooking meals, praying for you or just being with you.

- Make peace with God.

It's sometimes hard not to question or be angry at God when an adoption fails, especially after experiencing infertility as well. God knows your hurt and wants to help heal your pain—let Him.[22]

Other possible risks related to adoption may include unanticipated medical concerns and scant medical histories (which can especially be the case with international adoption). For children adopted from foster care and those who have been institutionalized in orphanages, there is also a greater risk of behavioral and psychological issues, such as attachment disorders. Many adoption experts say that, in most cases, these issues are not insurmountable with the right treatments, therapies, and parental love and support.

Can I Truly Love an Adopted Child?

When facing adoption, the question of whether an adopted child would be as wonderful or loved as a biological child can loom large. While not wanting to seem elitist or prejudicial and knowing that our hearts are capable of great love, it is still hard to let go of our fears and our desires to participate in the miracle of parenthood and creation.

One day while my kids and I were waiting in line, an older woman ahead of us started staring and the following conversation ensued:

> WOMAN: Are they all yours?
>
> ME: Yes.
>
> WOMAN: Your poor husband. So even the Chinese one is yours?
>
> EMMANUEL (who was almost four years old at the time): I'm not Chinese.
>
> ME (so proud that he spoke up to politely correct the antagonistic woman): That's right. You're not Chinese. Where were you born?
>
> EMMANUEL: In Vietnam.
>
> WOMAN: So he's adopted.
>
> ME: Yes.
>
> WOMAN: And do you love them all the same?

Me (gasp and cringe internally, and fight a growing desire to possibly hurt this woman, but since I feel strongly about needing to be a positive adoption advocate in the face of naiveté, I simply say): Yes, ma'am. Of course I love all my children the same. (By this point, Emmanuel has climbed onto my lap for security and is clearly not comfortable with the conversation.)

WOMAN (you'd think she would have let up by now): Are you sure?

The woman was next in line at that point and was called, so I don't think she heard my answer. Come to think of it, I actually can't recall if I answered her or not, but I know I hugged Emmanuel tightly and told him, "I love you very much." It was Emmanuel that I needed to remind that he was loved, not her anyway. Out of the corner of my eye, I noticed a sympathetic and incredulous nod coming from the gentleman standing across from us in line.

We get a lot of questions about our family, but that conversation is by far the hardest one we have endured. I welcome questions from strangers about adoption as I see it as an opportunity to challenge people's hearts and misconceptions about adoption, but to call into question my love for my children not once but twice in their presence was just plain inappropriate. At the root of her questioning, though, was a commonly held misconception that adopted children cannot be loved the same as biological ones. Perhaps some of us have those same fears that may be keeping us from entering into the adoption process; these fears are understandable and normal. Well, I'm here to say (and to shout it from the rooftops if need be) that, without a shadow of a doubt, one *can* love an adopted child as much as a biological one.

Biology does not guarantee love and attachment. The intensity of bonding and depth of emotion are the same, regardless of how a child joins the family. I'm not biologically related to my husband, but I choose to love him and he is my family. Why can't it be the same for an adopted child?

Truth be told, I did not take one look at Emmanuel when he came home at eight months old and fall instantly in love and instinctively feel he was my son. This does happen for some people, but it did not happen for me. But that also didn't happen for me at the birth of my biological children either! Love is a choice, and it sometimes takes time for it to grow. I also firmly believe that if God guides us to adoption it is because he also is giving us the grace to be able to love and nurture this child as our own, even if we didn't give birth to him or her.

Leap of Faith

So does adoption mean giving up on ever having a biological child; does it mean giving up one of the most hopeful statements, "with God all things are possible"? We would love clarity and a neon sign saying which road to take, but God does not work like that because he works through our freedom. Our freedom is a gift, and when we choose to give that freedom back to God, we are truly free.

Toward the end of his Spiritual Exercises (234), St. Ignatius places a prayer, commonly referred to as the Suscipe:

> Take, Lord, and receive all my liberty,
> my memory, my understanding,
> and my entire will,
> all I have and call my own.
> You have given all to me.
> To you, Lord, I return it.
> Everything is yours; do with it what you will.
> Give me only your love and your grace,
> that is enough for me.

Everything is yours, Lord. All we can do is act. For example, as a married couple aware of our fertility, we can make love during the fertile time of the month and be open to the possibility of God's gift of a new life, but we must also accept that the answer may be no. For couples who practice Natural Family Planning (NFP) and know the signs of their fertility, it would be difficult for them to not know if in a particular cycle the possibility of a pregnancy existed.

In the same way with adoption, we open ourselves to the process, to the possibility, and trust that he will guide us. In a way, this may be better; it means continuing to relinquish control.

Matthew and Elise said that infertility is the biggest blessing and gift they have ever received because it enabled them to adopt their three boys from Colombia. "Everything is perfect. The plan of God for us is perfect," said Matthew. "It has matured us and has enabled us to have our children. I see my children now and think it's impossible—we asked God for children and he sent us three. He's given us everything we've asked for and more."

My family and I can relate. In our situation, we were told we had unexplained infertility, but I have a pretty good explanation for our infertility: it was so that Emmanuel could be a part of our family. And so that this book could be written.

The "Prayer of Abandonment" for Adoptive Parents

Father, we abandon ourselves into your hands,
to send a child . . . or not . . . as you see fit.
You by whom the Word was made flesh,
send us a miracle, if this is what you desire.
Or lead us to her, if that be your will.

We do not ask for guarantees; no parent can.
Only light enough for the very next step.
We do not ask for a perfect child,
nor can we promise to be perfect parents.
Whatever you choose for us, whatever you desire
we abandon ourselves to your perfect will.

We are ready to offer our daily "yes,"
until that perfect will be revealed in us.
And until, at last perfected, we bear witness
to the work of redemption you began in Eden.

We love you, Lord, and offer ourselves to you,
wholly and without reservation.
We surrender ourselves, moment by moment,
knowing that this is only the first small step
of a lifetime of surrender,
so that we may be made more perfect in love.
That we might imitate, on earth as in heaven,
the redemptive love
the adoptive love
the selfless love
with which you first loved us.[23]

Adoption *Myths and Realities*

Myth: Adoption is outrageously expensive, out of reach for most families.

Reality: Adoption is often no more expensive than giving birth, depending upon your insurance. Costs to adopt domestically average $15,000 to 20,000 before the up to $13,170 Adoption Tax Credit the government gives and benefits that many employers offer.[24] Plus you can apply for grants and interest-free loans to help finance adoption. Is it cheap? No. But it's also not impossible. (See Affording Adoption below.)

Myth: Birth parents can show up at any time to reclaim their child.

Reality: Once an adoption is finalized, the adoptive family is recognized as the child's family by law. Despite the publicity surrounding a few high-profile cases, post-adoption revocations are extremely rare. It is vitally important for everyone involved—parents and children—to know that the birth parents have been given every opportunity to make the right decision and feel good about it. Less than one percent of domestic adoptions are contested in court.

Myth: Birth parents are all troubled teens.

Reality: Most birth parents today are over eighteen, but lack the resources to care for a child. It is generally with courage and love for their child that they terminate their parental rights.

Myth: Adopted children are more likely to be troubled than birth children.

Reality: Research shows that adoptees are as well-adjusted as their non-adopted peers. There is virtually no difference in psychological functioning between them.

Myth: Parents can't love an adopted child as much as they would a biological child.

Reality: Love and attachment are not the result of nor guaranteed by biology. The intensity of bonding and depth of emotion are the same, regardless of how the child joined the family.

Myth: Adopted children are bought.

Reality: The fees involved in adoption pay for such services as social work counseling and legal consultation—not for "buying" a baby, which is illegal around the world and in every state in the United States. All aspects of adoption are regulated by state laws and reviewed by judges who preside over finalizations to [ensure] that "baby buying" does not occur. There are possibly also fees for the birthmother's prenatal care in domestic adoption, as well as orphanage fees for continuing services to the children who remain behind in international adoption.

Myth: Adoption should be hidden from the child.

Reality: Though at some point the common thought was to hide from the child that they are adopted, this is no longer an accepted practice. It's not at all psychologically beneficial to hide the fact that a child is adopted. There are age-appropriate ways of addressing it but it should be done progressively as the child is capable of understanding the information.[25]

Originally published at www.adoptivefamilies.com.

Online Resources

US Department of Health and Human Services' Child Welfare
Information Gateway

www.childwelfare.gov
Features facts and information about foster and domestic
adoption

US State Department, Bureau of Consular Affairs, Intercountry Adoption

http://adoption.state.gov/index.php
Features information on which countries are available for
international adoption

Songs about Adoption

Steven Curtis Chapman
"When Love Takes You In"
"Meant to Be"

Michael McLean
"From God's Arms, to My Arms, to Yours"

Mark Schultz
"Everything to Me"

Patron Saints for Adoption

St. Joseph
St. Thomas More
St. Clotilde
St. William of Rochester
Blessed Teresa of Calcutta

Affording Adoption

Financial concerns are a huge obstacle for many people;
however, there are many grants and interest-free loans available for families desiring to adopt.

Adoption Tax Credit
www.irs.gov/taxtopics/tc607.html

The US government may issue up to $13,170 (in 2011) for qualified expenses paid to adopt an eligible child.[26]

Some employers have adoption assistance benefits to aid families desiring to adopt. Check with your employer to see if your job has any funding available.

Adopt Without Debt: Creative Ways to Cover the Cost of Adoption, by Julie Gumm, includes creative adoption fundraising efforts such as sales, events, auctions, and more.

There are innumerable funds for awarding grants to facilitate adoptions. It requires research and some paperwork, but it's worth it to be able to bring your child home. Here are just a couple:

Lifesong for Orphans
www.lifesongfororphans.org/adGrantLoans.html
   Interest-free loans and grants

Show Hope
www.showhope.org/AdoptionAid/Miracles.aspx
   Provides adoption aid; founded by Christian singer Steven Curtis Chapman and his family

What the Church Can Do to Support Adoption

Not everyone is called to adopt, but anyone can do something to help the world's 18.5 million orphans, recalling that we, too, are God's adopted children:

- Inform yourself. There are a lot of myths surrounding adoption, and it is our duty as Catholics who promote the dignity of all human life to be properly informed.

- Consider adoption as one of the fundamental life issues we rally around as Catholics. At times, the focus is solely on saying no to abortion, which is of unquestionable importance. But how do we actively support those who choose life through adoption?

- Be supportive of families who want to adopt, whether they have no children yet or they are seeking to add to their families.

Adoption can be a long and emotional process—ask them how you can best be of assistance.

- Consider assisting a family financially. Adoptions can be delayed because a family does not have enough money to bring a child home. Spearheading fundraisers after Masses (bake sales, craft sales, etc.), for example, can help parishioners who are adopting. Even if you know of no parishioners who are in the adoption process, starting a parish adoption fund to support adoptions (or to send to foundations that provide adoption grants) can be beneficial.

- Start adoption support groups in parishes and dioceses, such as the Elizabeth Ministry.

- Create awareness. Asking the simple question "Have you considered adoption?" could open up the possibility to couples who may never have thought of adopting before—or to women who find themselves unexpectedly pregnant and unsure of what to do. Priests, counselors, and spiritual directors who meet with couples confused by the myriad of illicit infertility treatments with which science entices them should also encourage couples to consider adoption.

- Challenge and encourage families to adopt from foster care (which costs virtually nothing) as well as children resulting from unplanned pregnancies, children with special needs, and mixed race or minority children—and then support them financially, emotionally, and spiritually.

- Pray for children who long for families, families who long for children, and women who lovingly and sacrificially give up their children in order to give them a better life than they can offer them.

Our prophetic voice as Catholics can help demonstrate that the adoption option is more than just a catchphrase—it truly is a loving option.[27]

> Be sincere of heart and steadfast, undisturbed in time of adversity. Cling to him, forsake him not; thus will your future be great. Accept whatever befalls you, in crushing misfortune be patient; for in fire gold is tested, and worthy men in the crucible of humiliation. Trust God and he

will help you; make straight your ways and hope in him. You who fear the Lord, wait for his mercy, turn not away lest you fall. You who fear the Lord, trust him, and your reward will not be lost. You who fear the Lord, hope for good things, for lasting joy and mercy. Study the generations long past and understand; has anyone hoped in the Lord and been disappointed? Has anyone persevered in his fear and been forsaken? Has anyone called upon him and been rebuffed? Compassionate and merciful is the Lord; he forgives sins, he saves in time of trouble.

Let us fall into the hands of the Lord and not into the hands of men, for equal to his majesty is the mercy that he shows.

Sirach 2:2–11, 18

Further Reading

Guarendi, Ray. *Adoption: Choosing It, Living It, Loving It*. Cincinnati: Servant Books, 2009.

We consider this a must-read book for anyone considering adoption. It has an easy-to-read Q&A type format and is written by a Catholic psychologist who, with his wife, has ten children, all adopted.

Wolfe, Jaymie Stuart. *The Call to Adoption: Becoming Your Child's Family*. Boston: Pauline Books, 2005.

$\mathcal{A}$ppendix
Resources

Ethicists

National Catholic Bioethics Center (NCBC)
6399 Drexel Rd.
Philadelphia, PA 19151
(215) 877-2660
www.ncbcenter.org
Father Tad Pacholczyk, director of education at the NCBC, is
the author of a column called Making Sense Out of Bioethics that appears in various diocesan newspapers across the
country.

Pope Paul VI Institute
6901 Mercy Road
Omaha, NE 68106
(402) 390-6600
www.popepaulvi.com; www.popepaulvi.com/
naproethics1_Home.htm

Medical Referrals and Resources

American Association of Pro-life Obstetricians and Gynecologists
www.aaplog.org
Includes a list of pro-life doctors that can be searched by area.

Apex Medical Technologies
(800) 345-3208
www.apexfertility.com
Nonspermicidal/nonlatex condom purchase for male fertility
evaluation (user perforates tip)

Broda O. Barnes Research Foundation
(203) 261-2101
www.brodabarnes.org

Gianna: The Catholic Healthcare Center for Women, New York
City and New Jersey
www.saintpetershcs.com/giannacenter/

International Institute of Restorative Reproductive Medicine
www.iirrm.org

National Certification Commission for Acupuncture and Oriental Medicine
www.nccaom.org
Acupuncture; L.Ac. after their name indicates a qualified
practitioner

One More Soul
www.onemoresoul.com

Pope Paul VI Institute
(402) 390-6600
www.popepaulvi.com
For infertility evaluation and treatment

Tepeyac Family Center, Fairfax, Virginia
www.tepeyacfamilycenter.com

Mental Health Referrals and Resources

Pastoral Solutions Institute
(740) 266-6461
www.exceptionalmarriages.com
For telephone marriage and family counseling

Saint Michael's Institute for the Psychological Sciences
(646) 424-0395
www.saintmichael.net

Nutrition Referrals and Resources

American Pro-Life Enterprise
(800) 227-8359
www.kuhar.com
Supplements recommended in Marilyn Shannon's *Fertility,*
Cycles and Nutrition available here

Green Pasture
www.greenpasture.org/public/Home/index.cfm
Provider of natural cod liver oil

International and American Associations of Clinical
Nutritionists
www.iaacn.org
Includes a searchable list of certified members

Optimox Corporation:
Phone (800) 233-1601
www.optimox.com
Supplements recommended in Marilyn Shannon's *Fertility,*
Cycles and Nutrition available here

Radiant Life Company
www.radiantlifecatalog.com
Wellness supplements including fish oil available here

Dr. Ron's Ultra-Pure
www.drrons.com
Provider of natural products

Standard Process
(800) 558-8740
www.standardprocess.com

Terms You Should Know

Artificial insemination with husband's sperm (AIH; homologous artificial insemination): Injection of a husband's processed semen into his wife's genital tract. Sperm can be placed into a cup, which is placed over the cervix. This technique is also used in artificial insemination by donor (AID).

Assisted hatching: An IVF technique of micromanipulation that uses an acidic solution to dissolve the shell around a two- to three-day-old embryo to improve chances of implantation.

Assisted Reproductive Technology (ART): Any procedure in which both eggs and semen are extracted from a woman and a man and manipulated with the intention of producing a baby.

Embryo: A fertilized egg that has begun the division process that will result in a fully formed person; used by scientists to refer to a baby until it reaches the fetal stage.

Embryo cryopreservation: The freezing of leftover embryos produced via IVF.

Fetus: Term used by the scientific community to refer to a preborn child eight weeks or older.

Gamete intrafallopian transfer (GIFT): Nearly ripe ova are obtained from the woman's follicles by ultrasonically guided aspiration techniques as for IVF. But one ovum, separated with an air bubble from a prepared seminal fluid sample, is immediately reinserted with plastic tubing into the woman's fallopian tube so that conception will occur within the body. Pregnancy rates are similar to IVF.

Heterologous artificial insemination (artificial insemination by donor, AID): Injection of a donor's (not the husband's) processed semen into a married woman's genital tract.

Intracytoplasmic sperm injection (ICSI): When men have low sperm counts or other problems, such as blocked ducts, spermatozoa can be obtained either by masturbation or, in the absence of a normal ductal system, by needle aspiration from the epididymis or even from the testis itself. A single sperm is then injected through the membrane of the ovum and the embryo cultured in the laboratory until it reaches the eight- to sixteen-cell stage, when it is inserted into the uterine cavity. Because the "natural selection" that occurs when sperm enter through the cervical mucus is excluded by this procedure, a number of birth defects have been recorded when conception was effected by ICSI.

Intrauterine insemination (IUI): Of "licitly obtained" (normal intercourse) but technologically prepared semen sample. The sperm are collected from a perforated condom after normal intercourse, washed, and then injected into the uterine cavity, bypassing the cervix to avoid "hostile" mucus. Cervical mucus hostility is an immunological reaction brought about by several known, and some unknown, factors. A postcoital test would find no living sperm in mucus during the fertile phase. Other treatments for cervical mucus hostility include abstinence for two years to allow the antibodies to diminish or disappear, or the use of condoms (not acceptable for Catholics). Various treatments with steroids have been tried without much success.

In vitro fertilization (IVF): Conception occurs outside the body "in a glass." Ordinarily, the woman is treated with hormones to stop her natural cycle and stimulated to ripen a number of ova. The ova are harvested from the follicle with a needle under ultrasonic guidance. The needle is inserted either through the vagina or abdomen. Ova are incubated in the laboratory with a carefully washed and adjusted specimen of semen to allow fertilization. Prior to implantation in the woman's uterus, embryos are examined in order to select the "best." Sometimes, one cell is removed for genetic testing. Usually, at least two embryos are implanted; in some centers, as many as four are implanted with the hope of getting at least one live baby. At times, three or four embryos thrive. Some clinics then offer the mother "embryo reduction" (selective abortion) to allow only one or two fetuses to develop further. Because the endometrium is considerably changed by the stimulation of ovaries to produce eggs, it is the practice in some centers to freeze the embryos and to implant them in a subsequent natural cycle. The disposition of frozen embryos varies with the wishes of the parents. "Spare embryos" may be preserved, donated to other women or to researchers, or destroyed.

Low Tubal Ovum Transfer (LTOT): When blockage to normal conception is found low in the tube, an ovum can be aspirated from the ovary and inserted into the uterus. The couple should have had normal intercourse during the fertile phase preceding the harvesting of the ovum. Conception rates are not yet reported.

Multifetal pregnancy reduction (also known as selective reduction): A euphemism used to describe the abortion of one or more children (at eight to twelve weeks) sharing the same womb. Unlike most abortions, the dead baby's body is resorbed by the mother's body.

Primary infertility: The standard medical definition of infertility is the inability to conceive after twelve months of contraceptive-free, targeted intercourse, but for couples who are charting (or women over thirty-five), the time frame is six months. The definition should also include mothers unable to carry any pregnancy to term.

Secondary infertility: The inability to conceive and carry a baby to term after doing so at least once before.

Sterility: A permanent condition inhibiting conception.

Tubal Ovum Transfer with Sperm (TOTS): An ART procedure in which semen is collected from a perforated condom (rather than masturbation) and placed with one or more eggs into a tube where they are kept separate from one another by an air bubble. The semen and eggs are then injected into the fallopian tubes. This technique is rarely performed anymore.

Zygote: A fertilized egg in the single-cell phase—that is, an undivided fertilized egg.

Zygote intrafallopian transfer (ZIFT): Ova and sperm are obtained analogously to IVF, but the zygote, that is, the newly fertilized embryo, is immediately transferred into the woman's tube with a catheter threaded through the uterus. This does not allow examination of the embryos as it would for IVF. The live birth rate is similar to IVF. Also known as pronuclear stage transfer (PROST).[1]

Notes

Chapter 1

1. The umbrella term of Natural Family Planning (NFP) refers to certain methods, accepted by the Catholic Church, that are used to achieve and avoid pregnancies. These methods are based on observation of the naturally occurring signs and symptoms of the fertile and infertile phases of a woman's menstrual cycle. See the appendix for a list of different NFP methods and where to learn them.

2. For couples who practice Natural Family Planning or for women over thirty-five, it is actually defined as six months of trying to conceive.

3. "Infertility," CDC National Center for Health Statistics, 2002, last updated April 2, 2009, www.cdc.gov/nchs/FASTATS/fertile.htm.

4. "Infertility Services," CDC National Survey of Family Growth, 2002, last updated July 2, 2010, www.cdc.gov/nchs/nsfg/abc_list_i.htm#infertilityservices.

5. Secondary infertility is defined as the inability to become pregnant, or to carry a pregnancy to term, following the birth of one or more biological children. The birth of the first child does not involve any assisted reproductive technologies or fertility medications.

6. "Infertility," Medline Plus, National Institute of Health, last updated August 24, 2011, www.nlm.nih.gov/medlineplus/infertility.html.

7. "Infertility/Fertility," National Institute of Child Health and Human Development, last updated October 20, 2006, www .nichd.nih.gov/health/topics/infertility_fertility.cfm.

8. "Outline for a National Action Plan for the Prevention, Detection and Management of Infertility," Centers for Disease Control and Prevention, May 7, 2010, www.cdc.gov/art/PDF/ NationalActionPlan.pdf, 3.

9. "Infertility," Mayo Clinic, June 24, 2011, www.mayoclinic .com/health/infertility/DS00310/METHOD = print.

10. "Infertility/Fertility."

11. "Infertility," Mayo Clinic.

12. Adapted from Hannah's Prayer Ministries.

Chapter 2

1. John Paul II, *Gratissimam sane*, 12.

2. "Prayer for Purity of Heart," Christopher West, accessed October 6, 2011, http://www.christopherwest.com/article1 .asp.

Chapter 3

1. "Assisted Reproductive Technology (ART)," Centers for Disease Control and Prevention, last updated August 19, 2011, www.cdc.gov/art.

2. Ibid.

3. Father Tom Knoblach, "Ethical Primer on Artificial Reproduction," last updated April 2005, www.stcdio.org/offices/ omf/natural-family-planning/achieving-pregnancy-infertility -a-reproductive-technologies/326-ethical-primer-on-artificial -reproduction.html.

4. Hanna Klaus, "Reproductive Technology Guidelines for Catholic Couples," United States Conference of Catholic

Bishops, 2009, accessed September 14, 2011, http://old.usccb .org/prolife/issues/nfp/treatment.shtml.

5. Jeannie Hannemann and Bruce Hannemann, *Infertility Journey: Making Faith-Informed Decisions Under the Guiding Hands of God,* booklet (Kaukauna, WI: Elizabeth Ministry International, n.d.).

6. Fr. John Hardon, "Artificial Insemination," Modern Catholic Dictionary, accessed September 14, 2011, www.catholicculture .org/culture/library/dictionary/index.cfm?id = 31983.

7. William Cardinal Levada, "Instruction *Dignitas Personae* on Certain Bioethical Questions," Congregation for the Doctrine of the Faith, September 8, 2008, www .vatican.va/roman_curia/congregations/cfaith/documents/ rc_con_cfaith_doc_20081208_dignitas-personae_en.html.

8. Ibid.

9. Klaus, "Reproductive Technology Guidelines."

10. Ibid. This process is detailed in chapter 4.

11. Ibid.

12. Edward J. Furton, "*Dignitas Personae* on Reproductive Technologies: A Commentary on *Dignitas Personae*, Part Two, nn 11–17," accessed September 14, 2011, www.ncbcenter.org/page .aspx?pid = 1007.

13. Christopher West, "In-Vitro Fertilization and the Hermeneutic of the Gift," accessed September 14, 2011, www.christ opherwest.com/page.asp?ContentID = 77.

14. Ibid.

15. John M. Haas, "Begotten Not Made: A Catholic View of Reproductive Technology," 1998, accessed September 14, 2011, http://old.usccb.org/prolife/programs/rlp/98rlphaa.shtml.

16. Katie Elrod with Paul Carpentier, "The Church's Best Kept Secret: Church Teaching on Infertility Treatment," in *Women, Sex and the Church: A Case for Catholic Teaching*, ed. Erika Bachiochi (Boston: Pauline Books and Media, 2010), 140.

17. "Human Embryo Cryopreservation," Georgia Reproductive Specialists, accessed September 14, 2011, www.ivf.com/cryo.html.

18. Hannemann and Hannemann, *Infertility Journey*.

19. "Outline for a National Action Plan for the Prevention, Detection and Management of Infertility," CDC, May 7, 2010, www.cdc.gov/art/PDF/NationalActionPlan.pdf.

20. For a list of other reproductive treatments, please see the appendix.

21. Hannemann and Hannemann, *Infertility Journey*.

22. John Henry Cardinal Newman, *The Idea of a University*, "Christianity and Medical Science: An Address to the Students of Medicine," 518, Newman Reader website, accessed October 10, 2011, http://www.newmanreader.org/works/idea/article10.html.

23. Jennifer Saake, "Prayer in the Face of Fertility Challenges," Hannah's Prayer Ministries. Accessed on June 3, 2011, www.hannah.org.

24. "Can Embryos Be Adopted? Interview with Moral Theologian Father Thomas Williams," *Zenit*, June 3, 2005, www.zenit.org/english.

25. "Life-Giving Love in an Age of Technology," United States Conference of Catholic Bishops, November 17, 2009, www.usccb.org/upload/lifegiving-love-age-technology-2009.pdf.

26. Levada, "Instruction *Dignitas Personae*," 19.

Chapter 4

1. Kathleen M. Basi, "Inside Infertility," *Family Foundations* 37, no. 4 (March/April 2011): 13–19.

2. Hannemann and Hannemann, *Infertility Journey.*

3. Elrod, "The Church's Best Kept Secret," 131.

4. Hannemann and Hannemann, *Infertility Journey.*

5. The websites for these organizations can be found at the end of the chapter.

6. Weston A. Price Foundation, home page, accessed September 15, 2011, www.westonaprice.org; Price-Pottinger Nutrition Foundation, home page, accessed September 15, 2011, www.ppnf.org/catalog/ppnf.

7. This prayer is often attributed to Pope Pius XII.

8. Fertility*Care*™ Centers of America, home page, accessed September 15, 2011, www.fertilitycare.org.

9. "Natural Family Planning," Marquette University, accessed September 15, 2011, http://nfp.marquette.edu.

10. List is from Hanna Klaus, "Reproductive Technology Guidelines for Catholic Couples," United States Conference of Catholic Bishops, 2009, accessed September 14, 2011, http://old.usccb.org/prolife/issues/nfp/treatment.shtml.

Chapter 5

1. Charles Shelton, "Discernment in Everyday Life: Spiritual and Psychological Considerations," *Spirituality Today* 34, no. 4 (winter 1982): 326–34.

2. David Lonsdale, *Eyes to See, Ears to Hear: An Introduction to Ignatian Spirituality* (Maryknoll, NY: Orbis Books, 2000), 108.

3. William J. Byron, *Jesuit Saturdays: Sharing the Ignatian Spirit with Friends and Colleagues* (Chicago: Loyola, 2008), 67.

4. One recommended book is *Discernment: The Art of Choosing Well*, by Pierre Wolff (Liguori, MO: Liguori, 2003). I found it particularly helpful, and it also forms the basis of this chapter.

5. The only exception to this rule is the person who is consumed in sin so much so that he or she is separated from God. In this case—and only in this case—the voice of God, which is grounded in truth and light, stings the conscience of the sinner, whose actions and way of life are completely opposite to the message of the voice of God—and thereby causes very troubling and disturbing feelings in the sinner.

Chapter 6

1. Suzanne, "Openness to Life," *Lear, Kent, Fool* (blog), May 7, 2010, www.learkentfool.com/?p=24.

2. John Paul II, *Salvifici Doloris*, 21, February 11, 1984, www.vatican.va/holy_father/john_paul_ii/apost_letters/documents/hf_jp-ii_apl_11021984_salvifici-doloris_en.html.

3. Mary Beth Chapman with Ellen Vaughn, *Choosing to See: A Journey of Struggle and Hope* (Grands Rapid, MI: Revell, 2010).

4. Holley Gerth, *Rain on Me: Devotions of Hope and Encouragement for Difficult Times* (Bloomington, MN: Summerside Press, 2008).

5. Emily Dickinson, "Hope," in *The Complete Poems of Emily Dickinson*, Thomas H. Johnson, ed. (Boston: Little, Brown and Company, 1961), 116.

6. "Prayer to Heal the Pain of Infertility," *Beliefnet*, accessed September 18, 2011, www.beliefnet.com/Faiths/Prayer/Prayers-Miscarriage-And-Infertility.aspx.

7. Adapted from Gerth, *Rain on Me*.

Chapter 7

1. Viktor E. Frankl, *Man's Search for Meaning*, part 1: "Experiences in a Concentration Camp" (Boston: Beacon, 2006), 123.

2. Margaret Silf, "Little Seeds, Little Deeds," *America*, November 22, 2010.

3. Hannemann and Hannemann, *Infertility Journey*.

4. Online Ministries, home page, Creighton University, accessed September 18, 2011, http://onlineministries .creighton.edu/CollaborativeMinistry/online.html.

5. Eddie O'Neill, "Catholic Women Struggling with Infertility Form Online Community," *Our Sunday Visitor Newsweekly*, January 9, 2011, www.osv.com/tabid/7621/itemid/7337/ Catholic-women-struggling-with-infertility-form-on.aspx.

6. Saint Gianna Beretta Molla, home page, accessed September 18, 2011, www.saintgianna.org/main.htm.

7. "Saints Anne and Joachim Novena," United States Conference of Bishops, accessed September 18, 2011, http://old .usccb.org/prolife/issues/nfp/nfpweek/Novena.pdf.

8. "Prayer to Our Lady of La Leche," Mission of Nombre de Dios and Shrine of Our Lady of La Leche, St. Augustine, Florida. Accessed September 18, 2011, www.missionandshrine .org/la_leche.htm. Used with permission.

Chapter 8

1. For Your Marriage, home page, accessed September 19, 2011, http://foryourmarriage.org.

2. Elizabeth Ministry, home page, accessed September 19, 2011, www.elizabethministry.com.

3. "Saints Anne and Joachim Novena," United States Conference of Bishops, accessed September 18, 2011, http://old .usccb.org/prolife/issues/nfp/nfpweek/Novena.pdf. Used with permission.

Chapter 9

1. This prayer is often attributed to Pope John XXIII.

2. Consult a doctor or nutritionist prior to taking any of these.

3. For a comparison of L-Carnitine and Acetyl L-Carnitine, compared to Proxeed™, see "Men's Fertility: Enhance with L-Carnitine and Acetyl L-Carnitine, Compare to Proxeed™," Discount Vitamins and Herbs, accessed September 19, 2011, www.discount-vitamins-herbs.net/mens-fertility.htm.

4. For information on male infertility issues, see "Male Infertility Alternative Treatment," HealthCommunities.com, last updated June 3, 2011, www.urologychannel.com/male infertility/treatment_alternative.shtml.

Chapter 10

1. Though neither Angelique nor Carmen personally experienced a miscarriage or stillbirth, many women around them had. The experiences shared here are the collective voices of many women.

2. See list of terms at the end of this chapter for definitions of D&C and D&E.

3. Colleen Connell Mitchell, "Soul Sisters: A Story of Joy and Sorrow," *St. Anthony Messenger*, June 2011, www.american catholic.org/samo/feature.aspx?articleid = 30&IssueID = 24.

4. *Shadowlands*. VHS. Directed by Richard Attenborough. 1993; United Kingdom: Paramount Pictures.

5. Current Trends Ectopic Pregnancy, www.cdc.gov/mmwr/ preview/mmwrhtml/00035709.htm.

6. It is rare that a heartbeat can be detected in an ectopic pregnancy.

7. Since funeral expenses can be high, the Knights of Columbus may cover the costs of funeral services in some areas.

8. *Code of Canon Law,* Can. 1176, §2, http://www.vatican.va/archive/ENG1104/__P4A.HTM.

9. "Instruction," *Donum Vitae,* I, 4. http://www.vatican.va/roman_curia/congregations/cfaith/documents/rc_con_cfaith_doc_19870222_respect-for-human-life_en.html.

10. *Code of Canon Law,* Can. 1183, §1-§2, http://www.vatican.va/archive/ENG1104/_P4C.HTM.

11. *Book of the Innocents,* prayer written by Susan Wills Committee for Pro-Life Activities, United States Conference of Catholic Bishops, 2003. Used with permission.

12. "Blessing of Parents After a Miscarriage." In *Book of Blessings,* by International Commission on English in the Liturgy, A Joint Commission of Catholic Bishops' Conferences. Collegeville, MN: Liturgical Press, 1989. www.catholicculture.org/culture/liturgicalyear/prayers/view.cfm?id-711.

13. Mother M. Angelica, "Miscarriage Prayer," *EWTN Faith,* accessed September 20, 2011, www.ewtn.com/Devotionals/prayers/miscarriage.htm.

14. Catholic Infertility Support Yahoo! Group, accessed September 20, 2011, http://health.groups.yahoo.com/group/catholic-fertility.

15. Some of the Catholic infertility bloggers have also experienced miscarriage and share their experiences on their blogs. See chapter 7 for a list.

Chapter 11

1. John Paul II, *Salvifici Doloris,* 28.

2. Ibid., 29.

3. Ibid., 29.

4. Ibid., 8.

5. Laura Flaherty, "Matt and Laura," Hannah's Heart Catholic Infertility Support Group, accessed September 20, 2011, http://hannahsheart.org/Matt_and_Laura.html.

6. Hannemann and Hanneman, *Infertility Journey*.

7. Flaherty, "Matt and Laura."

8. Emily Snipes, "Catholic Approach to Infertility," Diocese of Evansville, Indiana, accessed September 20, 2011, www.ourcatholicmarriage.org/nfp/infertility.

9. "Prayer to Blessed John Paul II for a Friend," Catholic Infertility Support Yahoo! Group, accessed September 20, 2011, http://health.groups.yahoo.com/group/catholic-fertility.

Chapter 12

1. Mary Ann Kuharski, "Adoption Is Biblical," Abortion Testimonials, accessed September 21, 2011, www.priestsforlife.org/testimonies/1143-adoption-is-biblical.

2. "8 Myths and Realities About Adoption," *Adoptive Families*, February 2005, www.adoptivefamilies.com/pdf/MythsAndRealities.pdf.

3. "Adoption Factbook Reveals New Domestic Adoption Study; Leads Discussion of Current State of Adoption," National Council for Adoption, May 24, 2011, www.adoptioncouncil.org/images/stories/Adoption_Factbook_Press_Release_Extended.pdf.

4. Ibid.

5. "Costs of Adopting," Factsheets for Families, Child Welfare Information Gateway, 2011, www.childwelfare.gov/pubs/s_cost/s_cost.cfm.

6. Levada, "Instruction *Dignitas Personae*," 13.

7. "Adoption Factbook."

8. Ibid.

9. "8 Myths and Realities."

10. "Costs of Adopting."

11. Ibid.

12. "Openness in Adoption," Factsheets for Families, Child Welfare Information Gateway, 2003, www.childwelfare.gov/pubs/f_openadopt.cfm.

13. "Statistics," US Department of State, Intercountry Adoption, 2007, http://adoption.state.gov/about_us/statistics.php.

14. "Adoption Factbook."

15. "Hague Convention," US Department of State, Intercountry Adoption, accessed September 21, 2011, http://adoption.state.gov/hague_convention.php.

16. "Costs of Adopting."

17. For information on the countries open for adoption with the United States, visit the US State Department's Web page on intercountry adoption, at http://adoption.state.gov/index.php.

18. Sarah, "Infertility: Practically Speaking," *Faith and Family Live!* (blog), September 9, 2010, www.faithandfamilylive.com/blog/infertility.

19. "On Infertility and Adoption," *This Cross I Embrace* (blog), May 4, 2011, http://thiscrossiembrace.blogspot.com.

20. "Question 52: May an Infertile Married Couple Try Tubal Ovum Transfer with Sperm?" *The Way of the Lord Jesus* 3, *Difficult Moral Questions*, February 1997, www.twotlj.org/G-3-52.html.

21. "On Infertility and Adoption."

22. Elliott Anderson, "Coping with a Failed Adoption," Adoption.com, accessed September 21, 2011, http://library.adoption.com/articles/coping-with-a-failed-adoption.html.

23. Heidi Hess Saxton, "The 'Prayer of Abandonment' for Adoptive Parents," March 31, 2008, *Mommy Monsters Inc.*

(blog), http://mommymonsters.blogspot.com/2008/03/prayer-for-couples-who-want-to-adopt.html.

24. This was the amount of the Adoption Tax Credit as of 2011 but this is subject to change on a year-to-year basis. The government can also repeal the credit at any time.

25. "8 Myths and Realities."

26. "Seven Facts About the Expanded Adoption Credit," *IRS. gov*, last updated March 4, 2011, www.irs.gov/newsroom/article/0,,id = 236174,00.html.

27. Angelique Ruhi-Lopez, "Opt to Adopt," Archdiocese of Miami, November 15, 2010, www.miamiarch.org/ip.asp?op = Blog_101112156793.

Appendix

1. Klaus, "Reproductive Technology Guidelines."

Angelique Ruhi-López has been married to Richard since 2003. They experienced infertility for one year before deciding to adopt their first child, Emmanuel, from Vietnam. They also have three biological children, Sebastian, Madeleine, and Anabella. Ruhi-López holds a master of science in theology degree from Boston College. She served as an award-winning staff writer at *La Voz Católica,* the Spanish-language newspaper of the Archdiocese of Miami. Ruhi-López is a stay-at-home mom, a freelance writer for *The Florida Catholic,* and a parenting blogger and web editor for the Archdiocese of Miami.

Carmen Santamaría has been married to Alex since 2001. They have two children, Monica and Antonio Javier, and two adopted children, Victoria and Daniel. They experienced more than three years of secondary infertility following the birth of their second child and continue to face this challenge. Santamaría received a master's degree in business administration and a juris doctor from the University of Miami where she served as executive editor of the *International and Comparative Law Review.* She writes and edits for the Association of Corporate Counsel and is a full-time mother and part-time attorney.

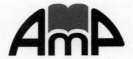

Founded in 1865, Ave Maria Press,
a ministry of the Congregation of
Holy Cross, is a Catholic publishing
company that serves the spiritual and
formative needs of the Church and its
schools, institutions, and ministers;
Christian individuals and families; and
others seeking spiritual nourishment.

———◆———

For a complete listing of titles from

Ave Maria Press

Sorin Books

Forest of Peace

Christian Classics

visit www.avemariapress.com

ave maria press® / Notre Dame, IN 46556
A Ministry of the United States Province of Holy Cross